Preparing for Weight Loss Surgery

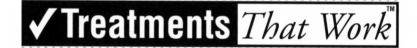

Preparing for Weight Loss Surgery

Workbook

Robin F. Apple • James Lock • Rebecka Peebles

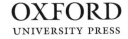

OXFORD

UNIVERSITY PRESS

2006

OXFORD
UNIVERSITY PRESS

Oxford University Press, Inc., publishes works that further
Oxford University's objective of excellence
in research, scholarship, and education.

Oxford New York
Auckland Cape Town Dar es Salaam Hong Kong Karachi
Kuala Lumpur Madrid Melbourne Mexico City Nairobi
New Delhi Shanghai Taipei Toronto

With offices in
Argentina Austria Brazil Chile Czech Republic France Greece
Guatemala Hungary Italy Japan Poland Portugal Singapore
South Korea Switzerland Thailand Turkey Ukraine Vietnam

Published by Oxford University Press, Inc.
198 Madison Avenue, New York, New York 10016

www.oup.com

Oxford is a registered trademark of Oxford University Press

ISBN-13 978-0-19-518940-7
ISBN 0-19-518940-X

9 8 7 6 5 4 3 2 1

Printed in the United States of America
on acid-free paper

About Treatments*ThatWork*™

One of the most difficult problems confronting patients with various disorders and diseases is finding the best help available. Everyone is aware of friends or family who have sought treatment from a seemingly reputable practitioner, only to find out later from another doctor that the original diagnosis was wrong or the treatments recommended were inappropriate or perhaps even harmful. Most patients, or family members, address this problem by reading everything they can about their symptoms, seeking out information on the Internet, or aggressively "asking around" to tap knowledge from friends and acquaintances. Governments and health care policymakers are also aware that people in need don't always get the best treatments—something they refer to as "variability in health care practices."

Now health care systems around the world are attempting to correct this variability by introducing "evidence-based practice." This simply means that it is in everyone's interest that patients get the most up-to-date and effective care for a particular problem. Health care policymakers have also recognized that it is very useful to give consumers of health care as much information as possible, so that they can make intelligent decisions in a collaborative effort to improve health and mental health. This series, Treatments*ThatWork*™, is designed to accomplish just that. Only the latest and most effective interventions for particular problems are described in user-friendly language. To be included in this series, each treatment program must pass the highest standards of evidence available, as determined by a scientific advisory board. Thus, when individuals suffering from these problems or their family members seek out an expert clinician who is familiar with these interventions and decides that they are appropriate, they will have confidence that they are receiving the best care available. Of course, only your health care professional can decide on the right mix of treatments for you.

This particular program presents the latest information on psychological and behavioral aspects of preparing for weight loss surgery and for sustaining weight loss after surgery while adjusting to the radically new lifestyle you will be leading. The program described in this manual has been developed by several of the leading experts in the world on weight loss surgery from Stanford University and includes a team of psychologists and surgeons. The necessity of this program is spelled out in the workbook, where it is noted that failure to change one's lifestyle and develop new ways of thinking about food and exercise could negate the beneficial effects of surgery and lead to substantially increased health risks. If you and your doctor decide that you are a good candidate for weight loss surgery, this program will help you to understand the various surgical options and, in working with your clinician, help you to adopt the lifestyle and dietary changes that will be necessary after surgery. In this program, then, you will learn skills to cope effectively with the necessity to eat smaller amounts of food more often, as well as to substantially decrease the intensity of the cues and triggers that have led to overeating or binge eating in the past and the emotional roller coaster that accompanies these eating episodes. To accomplish this, as you work with your clinician, this program will help you to change the way you think and feel about food and eating, and work to improve your self-image at the same time the pounds are slipping away.

David H. Barlow, Editor-in-Chief,
Treatments *That Work*™
Boston, Massachusetts

Contents

Chapter 1   Introduction   1

Chapter 2   Understanding Your Eating Behavior   9

Chapter 3   Normalizing and Keeping Track of Your Eating   19

Chapter 4   Weighing-In   27

Chapter 5   Pleasurable Alternative Activities   37

Chapter 6   Challenging Eating Situations:
             People, Places, and Foods   55

Chapter 7   Problem Solving and Cognitive Restructuring   69

Chapter 8   Body Image   77

Chapter 9   Congratulations! You're on Your Way to the O.R.   89

Chapter 10   What Happens After Surgery?   107

             References   123

             About the Authors   127

Preparing for Weight Loss Surgery

Chapter 1   *Introduction*

Congratulations on your decision to undergo weight loss surgery!

Perhaps you began to think about weight loss surgery after a conversation with your primary care physician, who was concerned about certain health problems that you have been struggling with that are related to obesity, such as heart disease, hypertension, high cholesterol, diabetes, or sleep apnea. Perhaps as weight loss surgeries of various types became more popular in the media, you learned more about one or more of the procedures and thought that some form of weight loss surgery might be right for you. Possibly, you've already had a friend or relative who has undergone weight loss surgery. Or maybe you just began to research it on your own after years of struggling ineffectively with more traditional methods for weight loss, typically involving dieting and exercise. In any case, your decision to undergo weight loss surgery represents an important step toward a healthy and active future.

You would not have opted for bariatric surgery if you weren't obese. In fact, surgery is not recommended as a weight management tool unless your body mass index, or BMI, is over 40, or over 35 with other significant problems affecting your health and quality of life. In the few studies that have examined weight loss surgery and compared it to traditional weight loss methods, bariatric surgery seems to result in greater weight loss over time in patients who are extremely overweight, rather than those just moderately so. Figure 1.1 shows the National Institute of Health's cutoffs for obesity.

Being overweight can affect almost every organ in your body. Table 1.1 lists most of the conditions that can adversely impact your health and are often caused or worsened by being significantly overweight.

Common Weight Loss Surgery Procedures

At this stage you have likely decided on the type of surgery you will have. Your primary health care physician should have gone over the various options available to you.

BMI	19	20	21	22	23	24	25	26	27	28	29	30	31	32	33	34	35
			Normal						Overweight					Obese			
Height (inches)									Body weight (pounds)								
58	91	96	100	105	110	115	119	124	129	134	138	143	148	153	158	162	167
59	94	99	104	109	114	119	124	128	133	138	143	148	153	158	163	168	173
60	97	102	107	112	118	123	128	133	138	143	148	153	158	163	168	174	179
61	100	106	111	116	122	127	132	137	143	148	153	158	164	169	174	180	185
62	104	109	115	120	126	131	136	142	147	153	158	164	169	175	180	186	191
63	107	113	118	124	130	135	141	146	152	158	163	169	175	180	186	191	197
64	110	116	122	128	134	140	145	151	157	163	169	174	180	186	192	197	204
65	114	120	126	132	138	144	150	156	162	168	174	180	186	192	198	204	210
66	118	124	130	136	142	148	155	161	167	173	179	186	192	198	204	210	216
67	121	127	134	140	146	153	159	166	172	178	185	191	198	204	211	217	223
68	125	131	138	144	151	158	164	171	177	184	190	197	203	210	216	223	230
69	128	135	142	149	155	162	169	176	182	189	196	203	209	216	223	230	236
70	132	139	146	153	160	167	174	181	188	195	202	209	216	222	229	236	243
71	136	143	150	157	165	172	179	186	193	200	208	215	222	229	236	243	250
72	140	147	154	162	169	177	184	191	199	206	213	221	228	235	242	250	258
73	144	151	159	166	174	182	189	197	204	212	219	227	235	242	250	257	265
74	148	155	163	171	179	186	194	202	210	218	225	233	241	249	256	264	272
75	152	160	168	176	184	192	200	208	216	224	232	240	248	256	264	272	279
76	156	164	172	180	189	197	205	213	221	230	238	246	254	263	271	279	287

Source: *The Practical Guide to the Identification, Evaluation, and Treatment of Overweight and Obesity in Adults.* National Heart, Lung, and Blood Institute and North American Association for the Study of Obesity. Bethesda, Md: National Institutes of Health; 2000. NIH Publication number 00-4084, October 2000.

Figure 1.1 Body Mass Index Chart

The means by which different types of bariatric surgeries work to effect weight loss can vary. Some are only restrictive in nature, thereby limiting the volume of food you can take in by creating a new, smaller stomach "pouch" and slowing the exit of food from the stomach (slowed gastric emptying). Others, in addition to restricting your intake, might also include a malabsorptive function. This means that the way food is absorbed, and the rapidity of absorption and elimination as the food moves through your stomach and then enters your small intestine, is changed by the surgery. Usually this happens because part of the small intestine is rerouted or removed.

Obese				Extreme obesity														
36	37	38	39	40	41	42	43	44	45	46	47	48	49	50	51	52	53	54
								Body weight (pounds)										
172	177	181	186	191	196	201	205	210	215	220	224	229	234	239	244	248	253	258
178	183	188	193	198	203	208	212	217	222	227	232	237	242	247	252	257	262	267
184	189	194	199	204	209	215	220	225	230	235	240	245	250	255	261	266	271	276
190	195	201	206	211	217	222	227	232	238	243	248	254	259	264	269	275	280	285
196	202	207	213	218	224	229	235	240	246	251	256	262	267	273	278	284	289	295
203	208	214	220	225	231	237	242	248	254	259	265	270	278	282	287	293	299	304
209	215	221	227	232	238	244	250	256	262	267	273	279	285	291	296	302	308	314
216	222	228	234	240	246	252	258	264	270	276	282	288	294	300	306	312	318	324
223	229	235	241	247	253	260	266	272	278	284	291	297	303	309	315	322	328	334
230	236	242	249	255	261	268	274	280	287	293	299	306	312	319	325	331	338	344
236	243	249	256	262	269	276	282	289	295	302	308	315	322	328	335	341	348	354
243	250	257	263	270	277	284	291	297	304	311	318	324	331	338	345	351	358	365
250	257	264	271	278	285	292	299	306	313	320	327	334	341	348	355	362	369	376
257	265	272	279	286	293	301	308	315	322	329	338	343	351	358	365	372	379	386
265	272	279	287	294	302	309	316	324	331	338	346	353	361	368	375	383	390	397
272	280	288	295	302	310	318	325	333	340	348	355	363	371	378	386	393	401	408
280	287	295	303	311	319	326	334	342	350	358	365	373	381	389	396	404	412	420
287	295	303	311	319	327	335	343	351	359	367	375	383	391	399	407	415	423	431
295	304	312	320	328	336	344	353	361	369	377	385	394	402	410	418	426	435	443

Some surgeries lead to more rapid weight loss and more complications. Some procedures are "open," meaning that they require a larger incision into the abdomen; some can be laparoscopically performed, meaning the surgeon (at some centers assisted by a robot) operates via a small camera that goes through a smaller incision; and some surgeries can be performed either way. The surgeries that are the best studied, most accepted, and most commonly performed are the Laparoscopic Adjustable Silicone Gastric Banding (LASGB) and the Roux-en-Y Gastric Bypass (RYGB). Some surgeons still perform a biliopancreatic diversion, although many consider this surgery to be on the decline, due to higher rates of complications and technical difficulties.

Table 1.1 Illnesses and Conditions Worsened by Obesity

Organ System	Illness	How Do I Get Tested for This?	Abnormal Levels
Cardiac	Hyperlipidemia	Blood tests	LDL > 130–160, dependent on risk factors HDL < 40 Cholesterol > 180–200 Triglycerides > 150–200
	Hypertension	Blood pressure reading	Systolic Blood Pressure > 120–139 or Diastolic Blood Pressure > 80–89
	Heart Disease (Coronary Artery Diseases, Heart Attacks, Stroke, Congestive Heart Failure)	Specialized testing, ask your doctor	Family history, abnormal tests, active symptoms, personal history of heart attack, stroke, or heart failure
	Metabolic Syndrome	Presence of 3 or more abnormal levels	Abdominal obesity, high triglycerides, low HDL, high blood pressure, high fasting glucose
Endocrine	Diabetes Type II	Blood tests	Nonfasting glucose > 200 + symptoms Fasting glucose > 126 2 hour glucose (after glucose load) > 200
	Polycystic Ovarian Syndrome	Physical exam, personal history, and/or lab tests	Menstrual irregularity and some sign of androgen excess (acne, extra hair growth in unwanted areas, overweight, and/or abnormal blood values)
Pulmonary	Obstructive Sleep Apnea	Polysomnogram (sleep study)	Abnormal sleep study
	Restrictive Lung Disease & Obesity Hypoventilation Syndrome	Lung function testing; polysomnogram	Restrictive lung function, buildup of carbon dioxide in the blood, excessive sleepiness, signs of heart failure over time
	Asthma	History, physical exam, lung function testing	Obstructive Lung Function
Gastrointestinal	Fatty Liver Disease	Lab tests, ultrasound	Elevated liver function, abnormal ultrasound or biopsy
	Reflux or Heartburn	History, physical exam, tests often unnecessary	Mild burning sensation in chest or stomach, acid taste in mouth after meals
	Gallstones	Exam, ultrasound	Periodic abdominal pain, gallstones seen on ultrasound
Orthopedic	Knee, Back, and Hip Disease	X-rays, physical exam, MRI when necessary	Abnormal range of motion, chronic pain, abnormal radiologic tests

Organ System	Illness	How Do I Get Tested for This?	Abnormal Levels
Brain	Idiopathic Intracranial Hypertension	Comprehensive eye exam, visual fields testing, lumbar puncture, MRI may be indicated	Persistent headaches, blind spots in vision, elevated spinal fluid pressure
Genitourinary	Stress incontinence	History	Incontinence while laughing, coughing, sneezing
	Gout	History, physical exam, lab tests	Joint inflammation, high uric acid level in the blood
Skin & Blood Vessels	Infections	Physical exam	Red skin with an odor, especially in skinfolds and creases: under the breasts, beneath the abdomen, in leg skin folds; fungal infections of the nails, poor wound healing due to poor circulation in the extremities
	Varicose Veins Deep Venous Thrombosis	Physical exam Physical exam, ultrasound	Dark purple veins on the lower legs
Cancer	All organs, but especially prostate, colon, breast, uterine	Multiple modalities	Abnormal test results

Table 1.2 offers a more detailed description of these and other less commonly performed procedures.

Working With Your Therapist

Now that you have made the decision to pursue weight loss surgery, you will work with a team of professionals who will help guide you through your surgery, both before and after it takes place. Usually, the team will consist of the surgeon, a physician, a dietician, an exercise therapist, and a social worker or other mental health professional. This team will work together to help you manage your body and mind as you notice rapid changes over the first year after surgery, and all members of the team are usually essential to long-term success. The different recommendations your team gives to you about post-operative management depend on your overall health status and the type of surgery performed.

Weight loss surgery is as "non-magical" as any diet or exercise program you have already tried, although it should significantly help you resolve your

Table 1.2 Surgical Procedures

	Name of Procedure	Description
Restrictive Procedures	Vertical Banded Gastroplasty (VBG)	In this procedure, the stomach is divided by a line of staples to produce a new gastric pouch, much smaller—only about an ounce in size. The outlet of the new pouch is similarly small, extending about 10–12 mm in diameter. This outlet empties into a section of old, larger stomach, which then empties as it used to into the small intestine. The surgeon usually reinforces the outlet with mesh or GORE-TEX to reinforce it. The VBG may be performed with an open incision or laparoscopically.
	Siliastic Ring Vertical Gastroplasty	A variant of the gastroplasty described above. Here, the stomach is again divided by a row of staples to produce a small gastric pouch. In this procedure, the new, smaller outlet of the new gastric pouch is reinforced by a silicone band to produce a narrow exit into the old section of stomach, as detailed above.
	Laparoscopic Adjustable Silicone Gastric Banding (LASGB)	This is a newer surgery, known as the LAP-BAND, approved by the U.S. Food and Drug Administration in 2001. It is only performed laparoscopically, as its name implies. Here, a new gastric pouch is formed with staples, as with the gastroplasty, but the band surrounding the outlet from the new pouch into the old part of the stomach is adjustable. This is achieved because the band is connected to a reservoir that is implanted under the skin. The surgeon can then inject saline (saltwater) into the reservoir, or remove it from the reservoir, in an outpatient office setting. This means that your surgeon can then tighten or loosen the band, adjusting the size of the gastric outlet.
Restrictive Malabsorptive	Roux-en-Y Gastric Bypass (RYGB)	The RYGB is the procedure most commonly performed and accepted. It involves creating a small (1/3–1 oz) gastric pouch by either separating or stapling the stomach. This pouch then drains via a narrow passageway to the middle part of the small intestine, the jejunum. This bypasses the duodenum, which food would normally traverse before arriving at the jejunum. The older portion of stomach then goes unused and maintains its normal connection to the duodenum and the first half of the jejunum. This end of the jejunum is then attached to a "new" small intestine created by the procedure above. This creates the Y referred to in the name of the procedure. This redirection of the small intestine creates a malabsorptive component to the procedure, in addition to the restrictive gastric pouch. RYGB may be performed with an open incision or laparoscopically.
	Biliopancreatic Diversion (BPD)	This surgery is considered more technically difficult and is less commonly performed. It involves a gastrectomy that is considered "subtotal," meaning that it leaves a much larger gastric pouch compared with the other options described above. The small intestine is divided at the level of the ileum (the third and final portion of the small intestine), and then the ileum is connected directly to this midsize gastric pouch. The remaining part of the small intestine is then attached to the ileum as well. This procedure thereby bypasses part of the stomach and the entire duodenum and jejunum, leaving only a small section of small intestine for absorption.

Name of Procedure	Description
Biliopancreatic Diversion with Duodenal Switch (BPDDS)	BPDDS is a variation of the BPD that preserves the first portion of the duodenum, the first section of the small intestine.
Jejunoileal Bypass	This surgery bypasses large portions of the small intestine; it is no longer recommended in the United States and Europe due to an unacceptably high rate of complications and mortality.

weight problem if you are compliant with all of the recommendations. While the surgery will leave you in essence with a "smaller stomach" that will alter the way you view food and the way your body handles it (e.g., feeling full faster, eliminating food more quickly, and possibly craving certain more healthy foods), it will ultimately be up to you to make the long-term surgical outcome—radical weight loss and weight loss maintenance—a successful one. What this will entail from you is a deep commitment to permanently altering aspects of your lifestyle that contributed to your becoming obese in the first place.

You might have thought at times that you were destined or doomed to become overweight. However, even if a biological predisposition to obesity was inherited from your parents, ultimately your eating habits and activity patterns have played a significant role. Deciding that you will make a commitment to eat healthfully and nutritiously and to exercise regularly is the key to ensuring long-term success with your surgery. Without this level of commitment to your future as a thinner and healthier person, the probability of the surgery leading to permanent weight loss maintenance is limited. If you can't honestly look at yourself in the mirror and affirm your commitment to making these changes and improvements for the rest of your life, your hopes and expectations regarding the surgery are likely to be unrealistic. These are the types of issues you will address in your therapy as you prepare for your surgery.

Throughout your sessions with your therapist, you will learn the skills that are required to adapt to the lifestyle and dietary changes that are necessary in order for you to sustain your weight loss after surgery. The treatment program outlined in this workbook is based on cognitive behavioral techniques that when used in conjunction with your therapy sessions will help you to develop a more thorough understanding of all aspects of your past and current problems with food and your weight. It will also help you to establish a regular pattern of eating, teach you about self-care and how to replace your negative eating habits with other, more pleasurable activities, and help you assume a lifestyle consistent with long-term weight loss maintenance. You will learn problem-solving skills and ways to change your negative thoughts about food, eating, your body, and yourself.

Chapter 2   *Understanding Your Eating Behavior*

Goals

■ To learn about the cognitive behavioral therapy (CBT) model for understanding the development of your weight and eating issues

■ To personalize the CBT model based on your own experience

■ To help you understand the way in which weight loss surgery is likely to affect these issues

If you are obese, that means that you have been overeating in one way or another, that is, ingesting more calories than your body needs and storing the excess as increased body weight or body fat. It might surprise you to find out that there are different forms of overeating—and that you might engage in some, but not others. It is important to identify the types of overeating problems that you have, so that appropriate interventions can be developed to address your specific eating problems. The following section helps you identify the types of overeating behaviors that you might engage in most frequently. Together with your therapist you will work to understand the reasons behind these behaviors, as well as ways to stop.

Types of Overeating

Overeating comes in different shapes and sizes. For example, there are binge eating episodes where you eat a large amount of food in a small amount of time, and in a way that is considered to be very different from the average person's eating experience. These binges usually lead to a feeling of being uncomfortably full or "stuffed." On the other hand, overeating can sometimes take the form of "grazing" throughout the day, that is, eating relatively small amounts of food frequently between standard snack or meal times, usually in response to cravings, boredom or other emotions, or the mere availability of food. For some individuals, overeating episodes are followed by a strong resolve to eat less, under-eat, starve for a few days, exercise more, or in extreme cases, to purge the excess food. Those who follow episodes of overeating with purging (or extreme or compulsive exercise or starving) on a regular basis are classified as having "bulimia nervosa" as opposed to "binge eating disorder." Most people who eventually become obese do not purge on a regular basis. If they did, they wouldn't be as overweight as they are. On the other hand, if you are purging regularly but have still managed to become obese, it is probably wise to delay your surgery until the purging behaviors are fully resolved.

Once you and your therapist understand the specific nature of your overeating habits, you can fit these into a larger model based on cognitive behavioral theory that takes into account other aspects of your lifestyle and current circumstances. This type of model will help you to better understand the interrelationships between your eating behaviors and weight, factors in your personal history, and current situations, thoughts, and feelings.

An Illustration of the Cognitive Behavioral Model of Overeating

Your therapist will discuss Figure 2.1 with you during your session.

The Cognitive Behavioral Model of Overeating

This figure (Figure 2.1) shows the vicious cycle of overeating followed by later attempts of various types to control eating. The CBT model of overeating suggests that there are specific links between certain eating behaviors, attitudes, feelings, and weight. For example, in our culture as a whole, most people tend to value, if not overvalue, being thin or even in some cases, extremely thin. The pressure to eat less felt by those who are overweight who also place significant value on thinness can be overwhelming and at times lead exactly to the behavior that is most unwelcome: that of overeating. For some, overeating in the short-term is quite pleasurable and therefore briefly combats the stress and depression that can come from the experience of being overweight or obese. In some instances, eating has become the primary tool for gratification and pleasure that overweight individuals have learned to use to soothe themselves in the event of negative emotions or problem situations.

Typically, after a brief period of pleasure, overeating can lead to negative feelings and thoughts about oneself and a feeling of failure, at least with re-

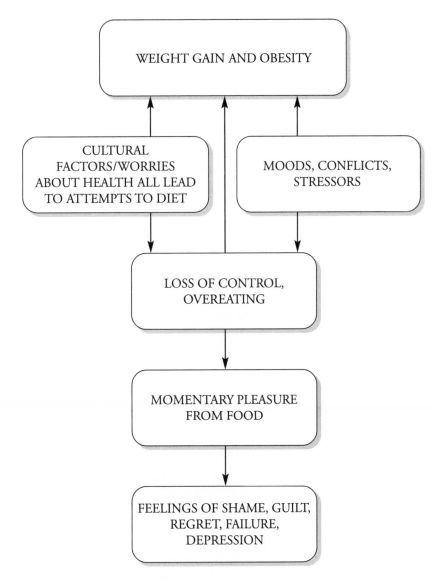

Figure 2.1 The Cognitive Behavioral Model of Overeating

spect to eating and weight control. While massive efforts to diet and exercise, even unsuccessfully, including hypervigilance, emotional energy, and "good intentions," often follow bouts of overeating, this extreme effort in and of itself can lead to feelings of stress and deprivation. That is, you may feel that you aren't "allowed," don't have a right to eat, or don't have access to the foods that you like. Frequently, these feelings can trigger episodes of overeating no matter what their source (e.g., actual or intended dieting).

In addition to the experience of deprivation, other aspects of one's life can contribute to having a lowered threshold for overeating. For example, general stress, intense emotions of other types, conflicts with people, and a distorted sense of hunger and fullness from a history of overeating and purging can create a situation in which it is impossible to clearly discern hunger and fullness cues.

Finally, there are often historical factors associated with overeating and becoming overweight. These might include the early experience of being teased and labeled fat, having been forced to diet as a young child, or retreating into overeating and weight gain to avoid certain challenges associated with growing up. In adulthood, overweight and overeating can often be associated with pregnancy, raising children, becoming more sedentary after starting to work again (or leaving a job), or being forced to give up certain sports or physical activities due to medical conditions or injuries. For some, excessive weight gain might be associated with giving up smoking, discontinuing stimulant drugs, or excessive alcohol intake.

You will want to spend a considerable amount of time talking with your therapist about all of the aspects of your life, past and present, that have played a role in your having become overweight, so that ample time can be spent understanding and working through the issues.

Your Life: Factors That Contributed to Overeating and Overweight

Using the form on pages 14–15, draw and/or write out a cognitive behavioral model that best fits your own experience with overeating and being overweight, both now and in the past. For example, you might start by first drawing out the factors that currently affect your weight and eating, and then noting a few of the relevant factors in your growing-up years or any other aspects of your history that affected your eating behaviors and your weight. Figure 2.2 shows a sample CBT model.

The Effects of Overeating: Emotional, Cognitive, and Behavioral

For many people, overeating—whether triggered by available food; cravings; negative emotions such as depression, anger, or boredom; conflicts with other people; or a desire to distract oneself by "creating" a new focus for negative energy—can lead to a variety of different outcomes. Overeating can be gratifying or uplifting in one way or another. For example, it can provide a form

It seems that overweight and depression run in my family. So I was overweight from a fairly young age. The problem seemed to get worse over time. As I became an adolescent and looks started to be more important, I retreated somewhat socially and started to eat as a way to make myself feel better. Obviously, this made the weight problem worse ... It has been hard ever since. Even though I have dieted a number of times, none of the weight losses that I have accomplished have "stuck" for more than a few months. Then when I started to have kids my weight just got higher and higher ... until the point where it seemed futile to try to do anything about it. Although I exercised in the past, with increasing weight it has been more and more difficult to move around, and for that reason I haven't done much exercise at all in the past couple of years, again making the weight problem even worse. So the surgery seems to be my only solution at this point.

Family history of weight problems and depression

Increasing weight led to decreasing physical activity and more weight gain

When I dieted I would feel deprived and then eat more as a result ...

Eating to feel better — e.g., to get over social isolation and depression

Diets didn't work anymore and frustration led to more eating and weight gain and lower mood.

Also stress of any type has usually triggered some overeating.

Figure 2.2 Sample CBT Model

A CBT Model to Fit Your Experience With Overeating and Overweight

of pleasure when there are few pleasures available; it can distract from difficult thoughts or feelings about any number of problem situations–in a sense it shifts the focus from one problem to another; it can provide a method for "acting out" or "breaking the rules" for someone who otherwise is quite compliant and sensitive to doing only "what is right."

Episodes of overeating are usually followed by a strong desire to control eating in the future, as well as a whole host of negative emotions, thoughts, beliefs, and behaviors about oneself in relation to having overeaten that develop fairly soon after the episode, even if the eating episode was on some level gratifying. These thoughts and beliefs might take the form of "I am going to be stuck doing this for the rest of my life," " I am never going to lose weight," or even more negatively "I am a fat pig" or "I am a loser." These thoughts and beliefs can generate an array of negative feelings such as: sadness, self-disgust, anger at oneself and others for having gotten into the situation in which overeating occurred, despair, and also probably a commitment to start dieting as soon as possible after the overeating episode is completed. For some people, overeating in the form of continuous grazing and consuming excessively large meals and snacks might not trigger so many extreme reactions but rather strengthen or ignite a sense of resignation and inevitability of future overeating and continued weight gain. In many cases, the negative thoughts, feelings, and beliefs also lead to compromised behaviors such as not getting out socially to visit with friends, feeling too full to do other tasks, or even additional overeating in an attempt to escape from the bad feelings.

Gastric Bypass Surgery and the CBT Model

Since the experience of weight loss surgery will change your relationship to food quite dramatically, you will also need to consider the issues discussed above in a different light. Mostly, weight loss surgery will help you better manage your reactions to both hunger and fullness (satiety). Specifically, after weight loss surgery of any type, you can expect to feel hungry less frequently and less intensely than before (for those of you who do actually experience hunger—some obese people do not). Also it will take much less food to fill you up once you do start to eat after becoming hungry, and your method of eating, which will involve taking very small bites of food, chewing them very well, and eating very, very slowly, will also increase the likelihood that you will feel full on much less food. Also, you will be given information about which foods to include in your diet and which to avoid and also strategies for alternating your intake of foods and liquids.

While, ultimately, the goal of weight loss surgery is to reduce your hunger level so that you can make wiser and less impulsive decisions about food, this surgery "benefit" can also come with certain costs. These might include the experience of deprivation that can accompany regular dieting when certain foods in certain quantities are restricted or the experience of being "left without tools" if you have used food as a primary means for coping with problem emotions and situations. Without replacing food with other positive and well-practiced tools for coping, any individual who is even enthusiastically attempting to restrict intake by choice can be left feeling unsettled, frustrated, deprived, or out of control. These feelings can lead to urges to overeat. Solutions for the problem of being "left without tools" will be discussed in a later chapter.

As you will discuss with your therapist, the reality is that even after weight loss surgery—which by now you should understand is no magical cure—overeating can happen, in one form or another. For example, you could find yourself unintentionally experimenting with creative strategies for overeating. These might include: frequent ingestion of small quantities of indulgence foods that are not ideal, such as very small amounts of sweets, candy, or peanut butter; taking in increasingly larger quantities of food, particularly once the new stomach pouch stretches some; or overeating deliberately on certain foods no longer digestible due to the characteristics of the specific weight loss surgery procedure that you had (e.g., such as fats after the duodenal switch procedure), thereby relying on the malabsorption syndrome, or "dumping," to in essence purge the excess calories.

The point being made here is that despite the surgery's "assistance" in controlling your eating, at least some of the fundamental features of the CBT model will still apply to your struggle to manage your intake. In your therapy, you will want to figure out in advance those areas that might prove risky for you. For example, after surgery, while you might not feel physically hungry in the manner that you did before, you might still struggle with physical and psychological cravings for particular types of foods or for food in general. Associated with these cravings may be emotions of frustration, loss, sadness, or even despair, for example the sense that you might never have the ability to consume any of these foods again or that you will always struggle with cravings to this degree of intensity. While the use of words like *always* and *never* signifies that you have been triggered into a cognitive lapse that involves clearly problematic and unhelpful thoughts, these errors in thinking can be addressed and modified using cognitive-restructuring procedures (discussed in a later chapter). By the same token, though, no matter how skillfully you might address the problematic thoughts, it is equally important to "get your behaviors onboard" so that you don't inadvertently contribute to any of the problems noted above.

Similarly, it is important to address any problem emotions you might notice in association with your surgery. In some cases, losing a significant amount of weight after weight loss surgery can in and of itself lead to the experience of excessive hunger, food cravings, and eventual overeating, as your body "fights" to reestablish its former "set point." Also, in some cases, negative emotions can accompany even desirable, radical weight loss and can lead to a pattern of emotional eating.

As you discuss your personalized version of the CBT model with your therapist and work hard to understand all of the issues involved, you will be able to more clearly ascertain the areas that need the most rehabilitative work prior to your surgery. No matter what, it is likely that one of the following chapters will address the issues that are troubling you the most.

Homework

✎ Read about and review the CBT model for understanding your eating and weight issues.

✎ Create your personalized version of the CBT model and discuss this with your therapist.

✎ Review the implications of weight loss surgery on the CBT formulation. If you are a teenager, go over your model with your parents and ask for feedback from them.

Chapter 3

Normalizing and Keeping Track of Your Eating

Goals

- To help you understand the rationale for establishing a regular pattern of eating

- To help you learn to establish a regular pattern of eating

- To educate you about the rationale for keeping food records

- To teach you a method for keeping track of your eating patterns using food records

The CBT model of overeating that explains the interrelationships between eating, thoughts, emotions, weight gain, and other behaviors and situations purports that the first steps toward making changes in this vicious cycle need to be taken at a behavioral level. For example, a key component in overcoming your problem eating habits or attitudes involves making a commitment to gathering more data about your eating behaviors by keeping some form of eating record. Another key factor involves establishing a regular pattern of eating, including keeping to a schedule of healthy, balanced, and not overly indulgent or overly stingy meals and snacks to interrupt any problematic cycles of overeating followed by compensatory undereating. Your therapist will discuss both of these principles and the following rationale in more detail with you in your sessions.

The belief is that prescription of a healthy pattern of eating can disrupt the strength of the links illustrated above (e.g., eating in response to triggers that include inappropriate hunger and cravings, emotions, the mere presence of food, etc.) that seem to dictate inevitable overeating. Disentangling these links and "cleaning up" your eating pattern by eating by the clock—on a regular but modifiable schedule—can help you free up your eating behaviors from inappropriate influences (those that aren't related to hunger or fullness). In this way you can slowly achieve healthier eating behaviors, as well as control over the co-attendant views of yourself and your weight that occur at times when you feel out of control or eat in an uncontrolled fashion. In many cases, too, this plan for regular eating can help you to slowly work toward your weight goal, since the pattern can help combat episodes of impulsive overeating.

The Importance of a Regular Pattern of Eating

As your therapist will discuss with you, the treatment of choice for problematic overeating behaviors that occur in response to triggers of any type, that is, hunger or cravings, emotions, available foods, and the like, has been the prescription of a regular and healthy pattern of eating. Obviously, the specifics of the planned eating pattern, the exact contents and quantities, will differ from individual to individual and will also depend upon the exact nature of the surgery that you are having and the recommendations of your particular surgery center. By and large, though, these recommendations tend to include the suggestion to consume three small meals and two or three small snacks a day (or five or six small meals) that are consumed not fewer than about 3 hours apart and not more than about 5 hours apart. The rationale behind this recommendation is that by eating in response to a flexible but predetermined schedule, nonessential and inappropriate food and eating "cues" such as those described above (e.g., emotions, cravings, the availability of food, and various interactions with people) will be washed out over time. The belief is that this mechanical style of eating "by the clock" will gradually become more automatic and natural, and increasingly will correspond to the ebb and flow of hunger and satiety signals, as these are progressively "retrained" through adherence to the schedule. In this way, over time, eating will be initiated appropriately albeit somewhat flexibly at meal and snack times, approximating the pattern that you will need to adopt post-operatively.

It will be particularly important after surgery that these meals and snacks be nutritionally dense (with particular attention to nutrients such as protein and limits on volume, as well as adequate fluid intake—preferably water or protein drinks—usually between meals). At the same time, healthy eating (in both the physical and psychological sense) must also involve some allowances for certain "small treats" that are at least somewhat indulgent. This will help stop problem cravings and deprivations that lead to out of control episodes of overeating. However, no matter what, the recommendation of a "normalized" relationship with food including the pattern and the contents and quantities remains the essential tool for getting eating behaviors that have gone awry back on track. In any case, the commitment to working "by the clock" in determining in advance just about when, just about what, just about how much, and just about where each meal and snack will take place, and sketching this out in "draft" form on a journal or log of some type, represents a very substantial step toward liberating your eating habits from untoward influences.

For Teenagers

If you are a teenager, there are some important factors that affect your ability to establish a healthy routine for eating. You may not control either the foods that are in your house or the times that your family eats. So, it is important that your parents and to a certain extent the entire family understand and accept the need for you (and to a certain extent, them) to change things. This will likely require that you and your parents meet together with your therapist to discuss how a structured eating program can be undertaken at your home. This involves identification of very specific obstacles—we don't eat meals at regular times, my parents don't cook, fast food is usually what we eat, and so on. Each of these will need to be addressed and solutions identified. Sometimes this will involve shopping with your parents for a period of time in order to make sure the right foods are available.

Using Food Records

The first step in trying to understand more about your eating patterns and your associated thoughts and feelings, and the contexts or situations in which you struggle with these, involves learning to record your behavior in journal form, using what is commonly known as a "food log" or "food record." You can talk with your therapist at length about your thoughts, feelings, and prior experiences with food records. Briefly, the food log is all about gathering data so that you don't have to rely on your memory alone to understand the details of your eating patterns, all that contributes to these, and how your weight is affected by the current patterns and any changes to them. When you complete food records, you also have a written record of your eating behavior that can be discussed in detail with your therapist during sessions.

A blank food record, along with instructions, is provided for you on pages 23 and 24. You may photocopy the record from this workbook or download multiple copies at the Treatments *ThatWork*™ Web site at http://www .oup.com/us/ttw. We encourage you to use these food records daily and to make your entries as close as possible to the time that you are eating. Of course, you can use the record to plan your eating patterns and specific snacks and meals in advance, and then cross-check to ensure that you followed through on your plan. Or you can make your entries after you've eaten. Either way, if done correctly, the food record can be an invaluable addition to your self-care plan around food. You will note that there are places on the record to document the time that you are eating, the amount and contents of food and liquid consumed, and whether or not you consider the eating episode to be a meal or a snack, to be "pro-plan" or "anti-plan" (essentially in control or out of control, e.g., "good" or "bad"), whether there was any untoward gastrointestinal consequence after, such as involuntary or spontaneous vomiting or diarrhea (or actual dumping syndrome) or voluntary vomiting, and what the situation or context was surrounding that particular eating episode. For example, where were you, who was around, what were you thinking, and what were you feeling as you began, progressed through, and completed the eating episode?

Keeping an ongoing record of your eating in this way will make it possible for you, together with your therapist, dietician, and/or your surgeon to really understand all that is contributing to and perpetuating your eating problems, as well as the exact nature of the problems. Without records, and left to rely only on your memory of what happened with food (given that eating tends to be an activity during which many people "space out," disassociate, or simply forget exactly what they were doing), it is highly likely that your recollection of your eating will be incomplete and inaccurate.

You might be quite skeptical about food records if you have worked with them before, perhaps in a structured diet program, while meeting with a dietician for consultation, or in some type of behavior therapy. Your reaction might be "this is not going to work—it never did before." Or you might feel as if keeping food records is all about "being controlled" by your therapist or the dietician with whom you are working. No matter what, all of these sentiments need to be explored with your therapist. Be forewarned that to succeed with this program you will need to transcend your tendency toward skepticism and trust that this experience with food records can be different, that is, that you can productively and therapeutically use these records to your advantage, rather than feel as if you are completing an assignment for someone else. But rest assured that regularly completing food records will be a different experience than any you've had before, if you use them as recommended in this program. Remember, if you want to really succeed with your food records, the best way to proceed is to make a commitment to recording your food intake (that means all meals, snacks, binges, or grazing episodes, as well as fluid intake) as close to the time of eating as possible. Any delay in your recording can lead to mistakes and, even more importantly, the experience of "disconnect" between your eating and what you later record in your food records. Again, you should raise any questions about the food records with your therapist.

For Teenagers

Sometimes teenagers don't like to keep food records. There is enough homework already, and keeping track of what you eat seems like a waste of time. However, it is important to try to overcome these hesitations. You will learn a lot about what and how you eat. When you are first getting started, you and your therapist will likely complete food records in-session to give you the idea and to show you how they can be useful. Sometimes, you may ask your parents to remind you to complete them. Over time, these food records will also be helpful when you meet with your other doctors to illustrate how you have changed your eating patterns and food choices. This will help demonstrate your commitment to lifestyle changes needed to support weight loss after your surgery.

Instructions for Use of Food Records

In the far left column note the time of the eating episode, then move across from column to column. Jot down the following: where you are at when you are eating, with whom are you eating, the type of food and beverage you are consuming, and roughly the amount that you are eating. Also, note whether you consider the episode to be a meal, snack, binge, or "grazing" type of eating experience, whether you ultimately purged your food in one way or another, and any related thoughts or feelings you had about this eating experience.

Food Record

Time	Place	Amount of Food and Liquid/Description	Meal, Snack, Binge, Graze?	Purge Y/N	Thoughts, Feelings, Situation/Context

The main point of food records has to do with this idea of staying connected to your own efforts to regularize your eating. The food record can help you track your progress on a meal by snack basis, thus reinforcing and motivating yourself to "stay on track" each and every step of the way. The record can also serve as a tool of intervention, stopping you in your tracks when you are at risk for lapsing into a nondesirable eating behavior, whether that is overeating at a scheduled meal or snack, skipping a meal that you have already committed to, engaging in "grazing" between set meals and snacks, or starting a process of negative thinking about food and eating that can lead to a downward spiral involving emotions and eating behaviors. Every time you are able to examine completed portions of your food log and note the number of success experiences that you have had, you can ease yourself back into "the groove" when you might have been tempted to feel negatively about your progress and give up. Similarly, as you become accustomed to using your food record in the moment, you can alert yourself to appreciating the number of options available at times that you are tempted to go off the program in one way or another, either by binge eating, overeating, or skipping a planned meal or snack. If you use your record in this way, as a tool of motivation and intervention, then you will be taking full advantage of the methodology. Your food records will provide an accurate record of your eating to your doctor, but they can be most powerful when you use them to help yourself with your day-to-day relationship with food.

Homework

✎ Review the rationale for maintaining a regular pattern of eating and discuss this with your therapist.

✎ Read and review the rationale for keeping food records and discuss this with your therapist.

✎ Review the instructions for use of food records.

✎ In your therapy session, set appropriate goals for the number of days you will record your eating during the next week.

Chapter 4 | *Weighing-In*

Goals

- To educate you about the rationale for and method of regular weighing

- To help you learn about the importance of other means for checking on and measuring your body weight, size, shape, and general appearance

- To help you understand the link between healthfully monitoring your body size and other healthy attitudes and behaviors

A Regular Pattern of Weighing

Most likely, you, your therapist, and your surgeon and/or your internist have discussed a regimen for weighing before your surgery that makes sense. For many, a weekly weigh-in session with a doctor can be helpful, so that changes in weight in either direction can be observed on a regular basis before too much time passes, in the event that any modifications (e.g., increasing or decreasing intake or activity) need to be made. If your weight is 350 pounds or above, it may be necessary to use your doctor's scale to get an accurate reading of your weight until it drops into a much lower range.

For many people with weight and eating problems, weighing themselves has been fraught with an incredible amount of stress and pressure, perfectionism, self-doubt and self-blame, anger at themselves or others, and a number of other feelings, some positive, of course, when the numbers are going in the right direction. Typically, these feelings have developed over time, in response to a number of dieting efforts that have been successful possibly for the short term but unsuccessful (as evidenced by your decision to undergo weight loss surgery) in the long term.

As a result of this level of sensitivity about your weight, including potentially becoming too upset in response to unwanted weight gain and "too excited" in response to weight loss, there is an overinvestment in what will be revealed by "the numbers" in any particular instance of weighing. And most likely that has led to your having developed certain patterns in the way that you weigh yourself, which you will be discussing in detail with your therapist. For example, some people who are highly vigilant and reactive to the numbers on the scale, and who use the numbers to define crucial aspects of themselves such as their self-worth or lovability, may check the scale daily or even more frequently (if this is possible, given their weight) to ensure that the numbers have changed, or haven't changed, or in any case to get a sense of "what the numbers are saying" about them.

The Risks of Weighing Too Frequently

A pattern of frequent weighing is problematic because it allows people to overreact to very small changes in their weight that virtually have no meaning at all. For example, shifts of one or more pounds in either direction that might reflect sodium or fluid intake changes from the day or days before can cause fairly exaggerated responses of either self-denigration or elation, both of which would be inappropriate given the predictable nature of those types of weight changes. These types of changes are more likely to be temporary and therefore not reflective of actual fat or lean body mass.

Avoiding the Scale

Some people with weight and eating issues have had such negative or emotionally powerful experiences with the scale that they feel unable to tolerate any relationship at all with "the numbers" and therefore avoid the scale at all costs. In some cases, even at physicians' offices, these people might ask to turn backward on the scale and request that the health care professional who is weighing them not even comment on the numbers. While this pattern of scale avoidance might in fact spare an individual with this type of extreme sensitivity some short-term unpleasantness or overly strong reactions, on the other hand it can, in allowing prolonged "distance" from the scale, contribute quite a lot to a person allowing their weight to change in the undesired direction (typically weight gain) due to the lack of reasonable feedback about what is happening in response to the eating habits that they have been sustaining for the period of time since the last weigh-in.

Avoiding the scale for too long can lead to an actual fear of the scale, not unlike a fear of spiders or any other type of phobia. The numbers can take on an even more exaggerated level of importance, to the point where they seem extremely powerful in determining how the person feels about themselves on any number of levels. Typically a pattern of extreme avoidance suggests that the person has started to allow the numbers to mean something to them about their value as a person that extends way beyond the domain of eating and weight control.

No matter what the particulars of the pattern—one of overly frequent weighing or avoidance of the scale—these relationships to weighing-in are problematic in that they suggest an overly strong emotional attachment to the numbers that likely interferes not only with a straightforward and healthy pattern of tracking weight changes as related to your eating, but also with you maintaining an appropriate and not overly embellished relationship between your weight and your sense of self (e.g., worthiness, lovability, etc.).

Corrective Strategies: Weekly Weighing and Other Measurements

As you and your therapist will discuss, one helpful strategy to address problem patterns of weighing is that of weighing in on a regular and preplanned basis, such as once a week on a specific day, at a specific time. Weighing regularly in this manner also is the best method for obtaining accurate comparison data week to week. This strategy can work for those who have been weighing too frequently, by cutting into this pattern in a very deliberate way. For example, once the day and time for weighing are selected, the scale can be deemed off-limits either by having it put into a closet or other hard-to-reach place or by limiting access to it by taking out the batteries or hanging a sign or "do not cross" rope as a reminder and a motivator to stay away from the scale on the other days. Or if the excessive weighing has been done in some other setting, problem solving and motivational exercises (e.g., analyzing costs and benefits) pertaining to limiting visits to that place to the weigh-in day can help. In addition, relaxation, distraction, and cognitive-restructuring methods might be useful in addressing any experience of anxiety or other problem mood states that occur on the days when weighing-in is no longer an option.

The strategy of committing to a specific day and time also applies to those who have been "scale avoiders." For those individuals, it may be necessary to either purchase an appropriate scale for the home or identify an alternative location (such as the doctor's office) where the scale can be easily accessed once a week on a specific day and at a specific time. For this group, weekly weighing-in might also need to be supplemented with problem-solving strategies of one type or another, relaxation exercises (to combat anxiety that occurs before, during, and possibly even after the weigh-in), and cognitive-restructuring exercises to combat any extreme or distorted thoughts that accompany the sight of "the numbers." (See chapter 7 and chapter 9 on cognitive-restructuring procedures, problem-solving techniques, and relaxation exercises.)

A weekly weight chart can help you maintain a visual image of your progress toward weight loss. In your session with your therapist, you can set up your weight graph (see page 31) in a form that will be most helpful to you.

Other indicators of body size and shape can also help you to work through your sensitivities and problem behaviors with the scale. These include the obvious, like how certain pieces of your clothing fit and how you fit into seats (whether at home, at work, in a movie theater, or on an airplane). You may also use a tape measure to measure various parts of your body, as well as obtain measurements of your body composition (e.g., percentages of lean body mass and fat). An indirect measure of your weight loss is an increase in your stamina when doing any number of physical activities, including exercise and incidentals such as walking up the stairs. It can be helpful to record some of this data over time, as well as your perceptions of these changes, in a log similar to your food records. Keeping a record of compliments that you receive pertaining to your weight loss can also be helpful and inspiring.

How Your Clothes Fit

Another very simple and easy way to figure out whether or not you're losing weight is to try on various items of clothing to determine their fit. If they are becoming looser, you're losing weight; if they are becoming tighter, you're gaining.

Weight Graph

Note: You can either use this 20 × 30 cell graph to track your weight over a 30-day period (e.g., a month), or you can otherwise assign meaningful numbers to the cells (e.g., each cell representing 1 week or 5 pounds) to keep track of your weight.

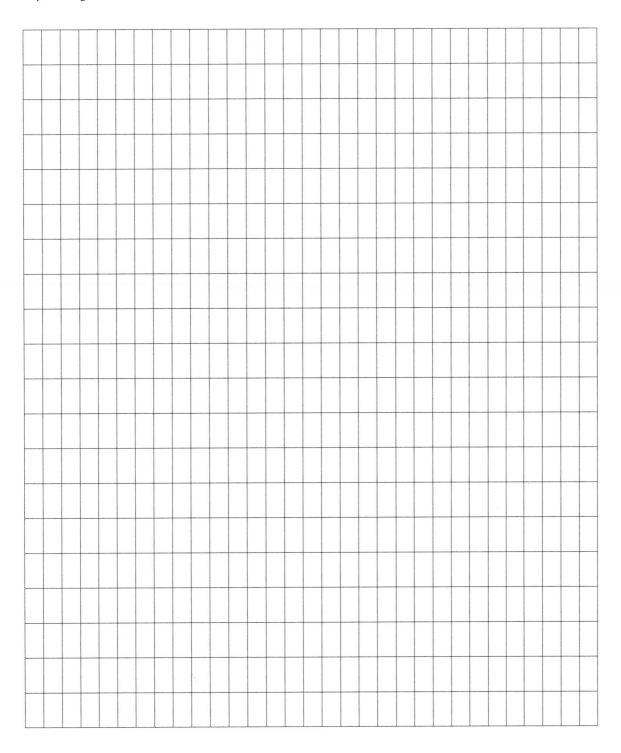

How the Furniture Fits You

This is another very simple way of tracking changes in your body. Over time, you will quickly find that you are much more easily fitting into seats, chairs, and other furniture that proved difficult for you in the past.

Taking Measurements

Another option for tracking your bodily changes separate from the scale involves using a tape measure to measure various parts of your body (the obvious choices being waist, hips, bust, upper arm, thigh, etc.). This method can be effective in offering you additional information about the changes your body is going through, as long as you measure accurately. It can be difficult to always get the correct or exact same spot, so you might have to practice or ask for some assistance from a significant other or your dietician if the results of your measurements seem "off" in any way.

Changes in Body Composition: Percentages of Fat and Lean Body Mass

These days, it is not difficult to find scales that measure body fat (although the accuracy of some of these might be questionable). Even better would be locating a gym or health club that offers body composition testing using calipers, underwater weighing, or other more sophisticated techniques. Finally, your surgeon, dietician, or internist might also have access to the most state-of-the-art techniques for tracking body composition over time as you lose weight.

Food Records

These records, discussed in the last chapter, ultimately will tell you everything you need to know, in that if you are maintaining a caloric intake or food plan that is providing less energy than your body needs, you will lose weight. By focusing on completing daily food records and examining your actual behaviors, including intake and the output of exercise, as opposed to the outcomes (as represented by the numbers on the scale), you will feel more empowered recognizing that what you do has an impact on the outcome.

Ease in Moving Around

Keeping track of either how long you are able to engage in a certain activity, such as treadmill walking or swimming laps, or rating your level of exertion while doing an activity can provide another helpful measure of how your weight loss and level of conditioning is progressing.

Compliments

When losing weight, it can be on the one hand uncomfortable to be noticed more than before or to be on the receiving end of a lot of compliments about your weight loss. But often it is these external sources of feedback (not unlike the scale, to some extent) that can help a person work through distortions they might have in their own perceptions of their weight. Obviously, you should not rely on compliments as the only source of pride-generating thoughts and feelings; in the end, you should serve as the primary source of enthusiastic feedback for yourself. However, in a "pinch" or a low spot, others' reactions can help you bridge the gap from feeling low to feeling better. Keep in mind, also, that in our culture of sensitivity to weight issues, some people may be reluctant to say much of anything at all about your weight loss for a very long time (until it is very obvious and visible).

Do not let the absence of compliments get you down, as you never know what is going on for other people in terms of their perceiving, but not commenting on, the transformation that is taking place. Also, you might find that you experience a range of reactions to others' compliments about your weight, from feeling proud and grateful for the acknowledgement to feeling shy, overly exposed, intruded upon, or even skeptical at times about what is being said (this is common when you don't yet feel your weight loss in the way others see it). Keep in mind also that it can be hard to know how to respond to compliments and questions about your weight loss that may come up at the same time. Remember that you are never under an obligation to fully explain anything about how you achieved your weight loss to anyone who does not know about your surgery. An explanation that can suffice in many different situations is "I made a commitment to eat healthy and exercise more!" In the end, those behaviors will be the optimal result of your having undergone the surgery.

Appearance and Weight Compliments Log

Date	Source	Positive Comments

The Appearance and Weight Compliments Log opposite provides a space for you to document the dates and types of compliments that you get from others regarding your weight as it changes. (In a later chapter, there will be a broader discussion of body image.)

It is important to use at least a few of the aforementioned approaches for measuring your weight loss before surgery on a weekly basis (except for others' compliments, which you can't control the frequency of). Write about them in a log, similar to your food record, so that you can review changes over time, rather than rely on your memory. You may want to use some of the more complicated methods, such as measuring body parts, once a month. Your food journal includes a space at the bottom to record your weight and also a section that can be used to note other body measurements.

Homework

✎ Find a place where you can weigh in regularly.

✎ Begin to document your weight on your Weight Graph.

✎ Read and think about the other issues presented in this chapter.

✎ Begin to make entries in your Appearance and Weight Compliments Log.

Chapter 5 | *Pleasurable Alternative Activities*

Goals

- To learn about the importance of pleasurable alternative behaviors that don't involve food and eating

- To make a list of these activities, those that can be used "in a pinch" and those that require more planning

- To understand more about issues of self-care in general and to work to improve your self-care regimen

When Eating Has Been the "Pleasure of Choice"

You will probably at some point discuss with your therapist the fact that for you eating may have become over time a primary form of pleasure and enjoyment that has always seemed to be available and literally "at your fingertips." You may have lapsed into a pattern of relying on food to give you pleasure because you lost touch with other interesting, creative, fun, and energetic activities that you might have engaged in with enthusiasm in the past. Perhaps you began not only to avoid certain activities but also to avoid people and social situations in general, due to shame or embarrassment about your weight.

In addition, you may have experienced certain emotions that may or may not have been primarily related to your weight, including depression, anxiety, or unpredictable mood states, that might have lifted temporarily when you ate something. As you might know, food can briefly and to some extent affect your brain chemistry in the same way that certain antidepressants do. Sometimes, even intense, positive emotions might have triggered an urge to eat, since eating can provide a form of distraction or can serve as an anesthetic by calming and soothing you in response to any form of arousal.

On the other hand, you might believe that you are simply a person who loves to eat, and you might attribute any or all of your overeating behaviors to a fondness for food. This view of food and eating might stem in part from your experiences as part of a certain community, family, or social group whose relationships revolved to a great extent around the experience of eating. You might also be someone who, in spite of eating a lot much of the time, never really felt full. You might have experienced hunger or strong cravings for food despite knowing that your appetite for eating was not reflective of a real need for more food. There are some people who ultimately end up overeating because food "takes over" where some type of substance abuse leaves off. You might be someone who fought hard to withdraw from addictions to other substances, such as alcohol or drugs, only to find that whatever was driving you to use these substances resurfaced—with a vengeance— in the form of your appetite and motivation for food and eating. Finally, since many of those who have struggled with weight and eating issues are "model citizens" in so many other areas of their lives, overeating for you may have represented one of the only opportunities to rebel without allowing others to control or dictate your actions and without very extreme consequences (aside from your obesity and all that accompanies it).

Why Does Eating Food Feel So Good?

While you may be extremely frustrated about your weight and your relationship to food and eating, it is likely that by this time food is also strongly associated with the experience of easy pleasure. It may be to the point that few if any alternatives feel quite as good, even if you push yourself to give other options a try. (And, truthfully, it may be that no other activity will ever feel quite as good, or as simple as food has, no matter how hard you try.) Nevertheless, in order to overcome your weight and eating problems, it is essential to stay focused on the importance of replacing your relationship with food with other pleasurable and meaningful activities that don't involve food. As your therapist will discuss with you, these activities will have to become part of your lifestyle and your coping repertoire, even if they don't feel particularly great or "do the trick" for you initially. The idea here is that with time, practice, and experimentation, these activities will become more and more like second nature to you, in the same way that your new and more healthy eating habits and exercise routines will become automatic. These alternative and pleasurable activities will not only serve to enrich your life away from food but will also be available to you in a pinch when you feel at risk for overeating for any reason and in need of some quick tools that can help you cope without giving in to the urges to eat.

Physical Activities May Be Best

Many people combating food problems report that initially their efforts to find other activities to replace the comfort, stimulation, distraction, and so forth that accompanied eating are most effective when these alternative activities involve physical movement as opposed to being sedentary in nature. Why would this be so? Usually, when people are motivated to eat, it is to find some method for stimulating themselves, whether to rev up, calm down, or numb out. After all, eating is itself a physical activity that has a variety of effects on all aspects of the body, from the brain on down. It makes sense then that to replace eating as the source of the stimulation, other physical activities would work best, certainly better than stationary activities such as watching TV at home (which by all accounts can be linked to a pattern of overeating and weight gain).

Some of the following physical activities are known to be helpful:

- Taking a hot shower or bubble bath

- Going for a walk or participating in some other type of exercise

- Getting a manicure

- Giving yourself a facial

- Working in the garden

- Engaging in sexual relations

- Going shopping (but not for food!)

Activities That Are Incompatible With Eating

In addition to requiring some energy output, most of the activities listed above are physically impossible to do while eating (or at least would make eating difficult). When trying out some new forms of pleasure activities, it is important not to allow them to become paired with eating cues. That means not eating while you're engaged in them. The reason for this is that once a given activity includes eating, it can send a signal that you should be eating every time you do it. For example, if you have been one to go to a lot of drive-through restaurants, you might notice a desire to "drive by and pick up something to eat" whether or not you are hungry, every time you are in the vicinity. Similarly, if there is a certain vending machine at work from which you buy a snack every afternoon at 2 P.M., you might find it quite difficult, if not impossible, to pass by without purchasing anything.

Getting Out of the House

While it is not always possible to leave your home to do something distracting and pleasurable in order to avoid overeating, it is helpful to do so if you are feeling tempted to overeat and you are at home alone with stocks of tempting foods (or even not-so-tempting foods). Going out may even involve the decision to get something (small and healthy) to eat as a compromise position as you consider the various options that you have. Still, this would be much better than running the risk of overindulging at home, where there may be large amounts of food and no particular controls (such as the presence of others) in place. Every time you experience a success in preventing yourself from engaging in an unnecessary overeating episode, you decrease the strength of the "pull" to eat for reasons other than appropriate hunger. At the same time, you strengthen your skill set for choosing more healthy alternative behaviors when you are tempted to inappropriately use food.

Realistic and Manageable Activities

It is important that as you learn to brainstorm about alternative forms of pleasure other than eating, you learn to do so in a way that is realistic. You need to come up with activities that you can actually afford, and do easily, in a variety of problem situations (e.g., at night at home alone, during the middle of a work day, on a weekend, or first thing in the morning– whenever it is that you feel at risk for overeating). For example, while it is nice to think about getting together with friends for a walk or an outing of some sort, people are not always available when we want them to be and don't always want to do what we want them to do at the times we're available. While it is probably beneficial to include some social activities on your list, as well as a range of activities you can do alone, you don't want to include only pleasurable alternatives that rely on others' company. Given that others are frequently unavailable, you could be left feeling frustrated and disappointed, and with those emotions onboard, possibly more inclined to turn to food for comfort.

"Big Ticket" Activities

While some "major" activities such as traveling or redecorating your home should be included on your list for special circumstances (e.g., when you have the time and money to work them into your life), these are best reserved as global lifestyle enhancers rather than "in the moment" strategies that can help you stay away from food. Similarly, if you live in a cold climate, certain activities such as outdoor tennis or golfing, while nice in theory and wonderful in the summer months, are not really possible during the winter months. Still, there would be nothing wrong with including these activities on your list as "distant" or "far off" possibilities to be used to enhance your lifestyle.

There are no set answers about what types of activities should be relaxing for any individual. The important idea here is to create a list of 10 or 20 things that you love (or like) to do that can help you to feel calmer, more at peace, relaxed, fulfilled, gratified, proud, and so on. The list might include some of the bigger ticket items that might interest you such as traveling to distant locations, signing up for a course on an interesting topic, redecorating a certain room in your house or apartment, or writing a short story or book. The list should also include several "in the moment" forms of pleasure that can be used "in a pinch" when you are feeling a rather immediate need to alter your mood state (or simply finding yourself with free time) without access to many of the other more serious endeavors. While the list will of course be individually tailored to your needs and interests, it might include the types of activities that are available to you, for example, in the middle of the day or at night, when no one else is around, without generating great expense. These could be reading a fun magazine or book; taking a hot bath or shower; taking a walk around the block; or engaging in breathing, progressive muscle relaxation, or imagery exercises (where you envision yourself taking part in a pleasurable scene of one type or another, etc.) Think of these relaxation and stress management activities as pleasurable alternatives. Use them in situations where in the past you may have too readily turned to food and eating to solve whatever mood challenges you faced at that time.

If you have had any type of substance abuse or alcohol problem (or cigarette smoking, for that matter) in the years prior to your surgery, creating a list of alternative pleasurable activities for relaxation is even more important.

Complete the form on page 43 to create a list of 10 or more activities that span the scale from "easy to do and very accessible" to the "big ticket items." This list ensures that you have ideas on hand, all of the time, regarding your next steps in taking care of your mood and state of mind (and also avoiding the choice of overeating as an option whenever you can).

Please use the following space to write out your list of pleasurable activities. Then post it in an easily accessible place, so that you are not at all at risk of losing your focus on these as options. Your therapist will help you brainstorm about the activities that might work for you, if you get stuck on your own.

Basic Self-Care

In addition to thinking about pleasurable alternative activities, there are several areas of basic self-care (in addition to your relationship with food) that you should thoughtfully consider and address as you prepare for gastric bypass surgery. Your therapist will discuss the basic concept of self-care with you and all that it means for you given your challenge of weight loss and your upcoming surgery. Areas of basic self-care include sleep, physical exercise, alcohol and caffeine, drug use, social and meaningful activities, relaxation and stress management, and of course your eating patterns.

Caring for Yourself in Addition to How You Eat

List of Basic Self-Care Tools

- Good sleep

- Physical exercise

List of Pleasurable Alternative Activities

1. _____

_____

2. _____

_____

3. _____

_____

4. _____

_____

5. _____

_____

6. _____

_____

7. _____

_____

8. _____

_____

9. _____

_____

10. _____

_____

- Moderation in use of alcohol and caffeine

- Abstinence from illicit drugs

- Engagement with people: social support and meaningful activities

- Other forms of relaxation and stress management (see pleasurable activities above)

- Healthy eating behaviors

While taking charge of your eating behaviors might appear to be the most pressing or essential of the important set of self-care components to work on as you prepare for your surgery, it may also be the most challenging. This is due to the basic complexity of your relationship with food and eating. Thus, these other areas that might superficially appear to be relatively more "easy" or straightforward to address are important to consider along with the changes you are trying to make in your eating. In making changes in these other areas, you will not only notice the benefits of the changes you make in these core self-care behaviors, but you will also begin to experience the type of mastery and success in following through with them on a regular basis that will generalize to the way that you handle your eating issues and such as you prepare for your surgery.

Sleep

For example, starting with sleep, it is important that you are trying as hard as possible to get 8 solid hours of sleep a night, if this is at all possible for you. Obviously the exact number of hours of sleep that you are able to get will depend to a great extent on your prior sleep patterns and your overall history with sleep, your current lifestyle, and any past lifestyle issues that might have affected the way that you relate to sleep. Whether you are at all close to or far from the ideal of 8 hours a night, it is important to keep the following ideas about sleep hygiene in mind, as you attempt to get your pattern back on track.

Sleep Hygiene Strategies (or "Cleaning Up" Your Sleep)

Many professionals in the area of sleep strongly recommend that you try to establish a regular bedtime and wake time. As with your food patterns, you should attempt to set your body clock to know just about when you expect yourself to settle down into sleep and just about when you expect to arise from sleep. And similar to planning a regular schedule of eating, it is also important for your sleep patterns that you decide on a regular place to sleep. For some, this may sound both obvious and simplistic. However, there are many people, particularly among those who suffer from sleep problems, who don't make the commitment or the effort to find their way to their own bed many nights, instead opting for falling asleep in front of the TV in the family room. In terms of the regular schedule for sleeping, let's say in reviewing your typical sleep patterns in recent weeks or months, you decide on 10 or 11 P.M. generally as your bedtime and 7 or 8 A.M. as your wake-up time.

Once these ideals are set, you attempt to establish a routine for bedtime and wake time that enables you to achieve your goals as straightforwardly as possible. This may mean setting your alarm clock to the time you would like to get up and including a remind or repeat function on your clock so that you don't let yourself off the hook by hitting the snooze button and going back to sleep. If sustaining a regular pattern of sleep is a new routine for you, you will probably need to establish a series of wind down behaviors and habits that will help you to feel de-stressed, relaxed, and sleepy when your actual bedtime approaches. These behaviors might include watching TV or reading (best if done in a room other than your bedroom), taking a warm bath, having a small snack (that is healthy and appropriate for you), doing mild stretching exercises, or engaging in relaxing visual imagery of some type.

Often, it is best to actually get into your bed only after you have become sleepy, not simply because you feel tired. It has been thought that exercising no fewer than 4 hours before bedtime works best, and consistent with the goals of good health and good self-care, regular exercise can often serve as a method for decreasing stress and tension and is therefore an aid to good sleep for most people. Once you practice with these concepts, you will understand and recognize the difference between how you are approaching sleep (and responding to sleep opportunities) now as compared to before. See Table 5.1 for a summary of sleep enhancement strategies.

Physical Activity and Exercise

The next self-care behavior to discuss is that of exercise. For most people, moderate, regular exercise is the obvious recommendation. It is important to remember, however, that your exercise goals and needs, and even the

Table 5.1 Sleep Enhancement Strategies

1. Decide on and commit to a regular bedtime and wake time. As much as possible, you should try to uphold this schedule even on weekends, although the tendency to "sleep-in" may necessitate that your bedtime is a bit later on weekend nights. The one caveat here is that if you find that you are not at all sleepy at your designated bed time, it can work best to continue your relaxation activities in another room until you feel sleepy enough to get into your bed (e.g., likely to fall asleep not too long after getting into bed). This way, you avoid pairing your bed with anything but sleepiness cues.

2. Commit to going to bed in your own bed in your own bedroom. This means, not falling asleep in front of the TV in the family room, or while reading to your child in his or her bedroom, or while reading in a lounge chair.

3. Both bedtime and wake up time warrant some type of routine that might include, for the former, "winding down" for a period of time (depending on how keyed up you generally are within a few hours of bed time) by engaging in relaxing and non-stressful activities such as: reading or watching TV (no high anxiety material, however!), taking a warm bath, having a small amount of warm milk, or ½ banana (if these are appropriate to your food plan).

4. Regular exercise can in general help a person to regulate their stress and relaxation levels and is seen mostly as an aid to sleep. It is important to remember, however, that exercise works best to enhance sleep when it is done no fewer than 4 hours before bedtime.

5. On the other hand, some mild stretching exercises, done shortly before bedtime might also be helpful. These could take the form of progressive muscle relaxation (e.g. starting with your feet and heading up to your calves, thigh muscles, abdominals, hands, biceps, face) and tensing each group for a count of 30 seconds, then releasing, before going on to the next group, with a 30-second tensing of all of the muscle groups together done at the very end.

6. Progressive muscle relaxation can also be combined with breathing exercises of various types, such as laying your hands on your belly and trying to take in deep, diaphragmatic breaths that are held for a few seconds each, particularly while envisioning some type of pleasant scene or experience (such as walking on the beach or lying on the grass).

way that you define "moderate," will depend upon your level of fitness and conditioning and the advice and recommendations of your medical team. Your team may have certain concerns or qualifications based on your weight, specific physical issues or problems, and your general health and fitness. For example, if you are extremely obese, have serious medical issues, have difficulty even walking around, and have not moved much for years, you may need to take it very slowly. It might be too difficult for you to jump into any type of regular routine, even a standard one involving 20–30 minutes of walking three times a week. The last thing you want to do is to push yourself too hard, to the point where the exercise you are doing is extremely uncomfortable for you, making it dangerous to your health and less likely for you to get back to it in any form. In your case, it might be enough to try to walk in place for 10 minutes at a time a few times a week either indoors or outdoors or to do the same 10 minutes of walking around the block (no hills though). Keep in mind that activities such as gardening, window shopping, and playing with your kids in the park all count toward your exercise goals; obviously any "up and active time" burns more calories than time spent sitting or lying down. In addition, "incidental" day-to-day activities such as parking your car further from the door or taking the stairs can add up to several more minutes of exercise a day—and over time that equates to a few more hours per week or month.

For those who have some lower body or extremity limitations, such as pain, stiffness, or certain joint replacements, making water exercise the primary activity rather than walking can help. Impact activities might aggravate pain, stiffness, or other pre-existing musculoskeletal problems, particularly those affecting the lower body. Also, general stretching activities, progressive muscle relaxation (e.g., first tensing and then relaxing various sets of your muscles at 30-second intervals, starting with your feet and moving upward to your head), and breathing training (e.g., engaging in diaphragmatic breathing, which uses the lower abdomen to support steady breaths that are blown out through your nose) can be considered a part of your exercise routine, as warm-up or cool-down activities. Discuss any new exercise routine with your medical team to make sure that it is within the guidelines they set for you. No matter what, creating a regular schedule and routine for your exercise, in a fashion that is similar to your efforts to regulate eating and sleeping behaviors, will help you to stay focused and committed to your exercise goals. Keeping an exercise log or journal, along with your food journal (or separately, if that seems better) can also be helpful.

Caffeine Intake

You are probably not accustomed to thinking of caffeine as a potential substance to be overused or abused. Excessive intake of caffeine can play a role in a person's experience of anxiety, stress, and tension, and can also contribute to the kinds of intense feeling states that can trigger episodes of overeating. While there are no very specific guidelines or absolutes pertaining to caffeine intake, it is a good idea to try to limit your intake to no more than a few caffeinated beverages a day. In terms of coffee, tea, and soda (although most surgeons specify that you are not supposed to drink many—or any—carbonated beverages following weight loss surgery), you should limit yourself to two 8–12 ounce servings of coffee and possibly an additional caffeinated beverage (such as tea, diet hot chocolate, or soda, if this is allowed for you) per day. The downside to drinking a lot of coffee is that it can give a person the "jitters" and a sense of incredibly overwhelming anxiety, urgency, or in some cases panic—all feeling states that for you may have been quelled with food, alcohol, or other nonoptimal tools for coping. Also, caffeine can dampen appetite in the short term while in the long term actually stimulate appetite by causing metabolism to speed up enough that one is left hungrier than he or she should be based on intake. One additional issue with caffeine intake, particularly when it comes from coffee, and instant coffee more than percolated coffee, is that of gastro-intestinal distress, in some cases diarrhea and in some cases gastric upset or heartburn.

Alcohol

Many weight loss surgery programs advise post-operative patients not to drink alcohol for at least the first year after surgery—while a small indulgence on occasion might be acceptable—and thereafter limit their alcohol intake as much as possible. The reasons for this are many. First, alcohol, while providing a lot of calories (200 calories per 8 ounces of wine, 150 calories for a standard 12 ounce serving of beer) provides no nutrition otherwise. The ingestion of these calories will contribute obviously to the overall calorie intake, without providing the necessary proteins that are needed to keep the body healthy. (Yes, alcohol will provide carbohydrates but in a form that contributes nothing else nutritionally.) Secondly, people typically are less thoughtful, clear, and committed to exercising good judgment following consumption of alcohol than they would be when not drinking. (Think back to times, if any, that you might have been under the influence, and recall what might have been some compromised behavior or thinking on your part.)

This lack of stellar judgment can even affect the way a person relates to food; that is, it can disrupt the usual "controls" that have kept your eating in check while dieting to lose weight before your surgery (if that was a requirement or recommendation for you) and since your surgery. You don't want alcohol to get in the way of your "using your head" in all matters, including those of food intake. Finally, alcohol is a substance, as is food, and in that way it can appear at times to be a useful and productive tool for self-regulation—that is, regulating intense emotions, longer-standing problem moods, or other bouts of uninvited "intensity" of one type or another.

While alcohol can have the effect of adjusting your emotions, it is far from a productive solution. If used for this purpose over time, alcohol can begin to parallel or mimic prior problematic use of food, which for many of those who have contended with food problems has at some level provided a self-soothing and gratifying component to their coping repertoire. Rather than replacing food with another substance that can be overused or abused, or one that can become addictive or habitual, it is preferable to use other strategies such as talking to friends and loved ones, or a therapist, or engaging in meaningful hobbies or work to move through the problem times. After all, replacing one addiction with another is not your goal! If for any reason you feel that alcohol has become a problem for you, for instance, if you are drinking every day and in a fashion that you are uncomfortable with, you need to address this with a professional as soon as possible. You may consider attending Alcoholics Anonymous (AA), which has an excellent reputation as a forum for resolving substance abuse issues.

Illicit Drugs

Much of the above discussion of alcohol also applies to the use of illicit drugs, although in the case of those, it is imperative that you seek help if you have experienced any level of use, not just use that has reached a problematic proportion in your life. Whereas a small amount of alcohol can be acceptable (once your surgeon clears you for this), no amount of illicit drug is at all acceptable, whether this be an "upper" or stimulant such as cocaine, methamphetamine, or any form of "crank," "crack," or "speed." If you have a past history of use of any one of these drugs, you would have had to report that you were clean for at least 5 years to be accepted as a surgical candidate. For those of you who used in the past, use at this time would represent a form of lapse or relapse that would signal the possibility of an ongoing use pattern developing once again. Whether this is the situation for you, or you are a new user of this type of drug, the issues discussed above with respect to alcohol would apply (e.g., using the substance to "replace" food for emotional soothing or gratification or losing the capacity for good and solid judgment once under the influence of the substance, including with respect to your food choices) and would require some form of intervention as soon as possible. Stated as simply as possible: there is no room for illicit drug use after weight loss surgery.

While there are obviously no hard and fast rules about what an adequate social support network could or should look like, the experience of having people in your life—who care about you and whom you care about—can't be overemphasized. Whether these people include a significant other, family members, friends, or an assortment of all of the above, staying connected to other people in intimate ways—through reciprocal conversation, shared activities, fun times and hard times—the existence of important others in one's life has been linked to decreased stress and disease states and overall sense of health and well-being. As someone who has been dealing with a very significant weight problem for some time, you may (or may not) have let your social life lapse into near nonexistence. If this has happened to you—out of sheer exhaustion related to your physical state, social anxiety, lack of opportunity, or on some level, a perceived lack of interest in relationships (that may reflect other emotional issues such as depression or low self-esteem or a sense of resignation and "giving up")—it is time to change all of that and restimulate your social life so that once again you feel as if you live among and along with other people.

One of the most straightforward and obvious ways to start this process is to take advantage of the network of people to which you are exposed through your involvement in one or more ongoing pre- and post-op weight loss surgery support groups. As a starting point at the very least, a therapeutic group experience such as this can help you retool your conversational skills, your feelings of safety around personal self-disclosure, your sense of understanding and empathy for others' circumstances, and your level of confidence that others will listen to you and take your issues and needs seriously. (If the latter does not seem to be present in the group in which you are involved, you should seriously consider changing over to another group, if this is at all possible for you.) Also, in the context of a weight loss surgery support group, you might hear about other opportunities that are social in nature, for example, in learning about the interests, vocations, avocations, or hobbies of the other members of the group. For example, if a group member volunteers at a communal garden, and gardening (or volunteer work) has been of interest to you, you might be able to make use of the group connection to get started pursuing those areas of interest.

Also, it may be that friendships that begin in the group might extend far beyond the group experience (although this may differ group to group, according to the policies and procedures of the given group that you are a part of) to include recreational get-togethers and activities that involve you and one or more other people. The idea is not to limit your socializing to members of your group but to rebuild your socializing muscle, if you have been out of practice for any length of time.

On the other hand, if you are someone who has been diligently maintaining a social life, with an array of people and opportunities for forming meaningful connections, the message here would be simply one of continuing what you are doing and possibly extending it somewhat. To either deepen your existing relationships, expand upon those that are currently active, or create entirely new relationships will involve taking some risks—that is, extending yourself beyond your comfort zone to create something new. While risk taking is never easy, it remains one of the essentials for changing one's life and creating something new, similar to what you have decided to do in pursuing gastric bypass surgery as an option to solve your problems with weight.

For Teenagers

As a teenager, your social activities are in part structured by school and related activities. Like many adults, you may feel that you will be rejected or teased by peer groups. However, you may also have a few close friends that you feel that you can really trust. It is important to keep those close friends while also beginning to reach out occasionally for new friends. Some of the best ways for you to find new possible friends is through after-school activities or through youth groups associated with your religious practices. The reason this is the case is that there are likely to be similar interests among members of these groups that can make the initial stages of making friends easier. Many times teenagers struggling with obesity have retreated to their families out of fear of humiliation or actual harassment. Although it may be difficult, you should work with your therapist to identify reasonable ways to work on new friendships. Building new friendships will not mean that you no longer need your family, but it may mean that you will feel less dependent on them. For most adolescents, this is a good thing.

During the period of time in which you have been waiting and planning for your surgery, and possibly even for some of the time when you were struggling with obesity, you might have disengaged from people and social activities, as well as meaningful roles and activities that you otherwise might have taken on enthusiastically. For example, perhaps you decided to withdraw from certain recreational activities that you enjoyed and added value to, such as performing in a musical group, having an active role on an athletic team, or taking on a leadership role at work, within a religious organization, or in a volunteer capacity. Since self-esteem and self-concept reflects the number of "eggs in your basket" (or the diversity of your meaningful roles and involvements with people and activities), it is important that you begin the process of rebuilding this part of your life. Opposite is a space for you to list some of the meaningful activities and competent roles that you have in place now and that you would like to work toward reinstating.

For Teenagers

Adolescents are first beginning to explore what things they would like to do and find meaningful. You might find participation in a youth group, volunteer organization, or extracurricular activity works well for exploring what interests and excites you. For many of you, however, schoolwork and preparing for college and work may be the main focus. You may find that by increasing your dedication to efforts that will lead to college or a career will help you to focus on the other aspects of your life that relate to changing your eating and health-promoting behaviors.

Homework

✎ Review all sections of the chapter and discuss these with your therapist.

✎ Create your list of pleasurable alternative activities.

✎ Choose at least one of the activities to do in a situation in which you feel at risk for overeating.

✎ Pick two or three of the basic self-care areas to start working on (e.g., improving your sleep and increasing your social network).

Meaningful Roles and Activities—Now and Plans for the Future

Now	Plan to Get Started Soon

Chapter 6

Challenging Eating Situations People, Places, and Foods

Goals

- ■ To help you identify the situations, people, places, and foods that are most challenging for you as you increasingly take charge of your eating and weight problem

- ■ To help you learn to identify the alternative situations, people, places, and foods that contribute to healthy eating behaviors and attitudes

- ■ To help you identify certain foods that have been most challenging for you as well as a method for becoming more comfortable with these foods

The struggle to gain control over your eating and to ultimately find a way to eat that allows for slow but steady weight loss pre-surgery involves many different factors. Obviously the choice of the specific foods that you eat and the portions you consume of those foods—both "good and bad," "healthy or indulgent," and so forth—will likely have the most pronounced impact on your weight, along with of course the degree of "output" (e.g., physical activity, such as planned exercise and "unintentional" movement such as taking the stairs, parking farther away, etc.) that you are able to fit into your schedule. Believe it or not, active choices that you can make about the settings in which you eat and the people that join you in those settings can also play a major role in contributing to the quality of your eating behavior in any one instance. Your therapist will help you identify the changes that you need to make in these areas to be more successful in your struggle to lose weight.

Stimulus Control: Eating in All the Right Places

When it comes to eating, certain settings are more appropriate than others. Obviously, the kitchen, dining room, picnic table, and breakfast nook are areas in which eating regularly takes place; these places are already steeped in eating cues and probably every time you sit down at one of them, you are conditioned to want to eat something. On the other hand, places like the couch in front of the TV, the bedroom, the bathtub, the work desk, in front of the computer, and the car are not typical locations for eating and are only paired with "eating cues" if you allow them to become associated with food by regularly eating when you are in these places. Once these unnatural eating situations become linked with food, it can be very difficult to disentangle them; that is, refraining from eating while watching TV will be incredibly hard if nearly every time you sit down to watch TV you have eaten something.

You might be laughing and thinking that it is quite unbelievable that others actually eat while in bed or in the bathtub, but this actually does happen and complicates things a lot when that individual then makes an attempt to "purify" their eating environment by trying to contain their eating only in the appropriate settings. Initially, it just doesn't feel right. Thus, the more quickly you can get a handle on limiting the number of automatic associations to food and eating by pairing eating only with the places in which it is meant to happen, the easier it will be for you to take charge of your eating behavior.

The first place to start is to actually take an inventory, first verbally with your therapist and then in written form, of all of the places in which you currently eat or drink something. You might have to really jog your memory here as some of these behaviors can become so automatic or unconscious that you might not even realize that you are eating in situations or places in which you ideally shouldn't. Use the form on page 57 to create a list of all of your current nonoptimal eating environments that have now become associated with food cues. The areas have been categorized into "home," "work," and "other" groupings to help jog your memory about what you are doing in the various settings. Simply check either the "yes" or "no" column for each area listed, and note any additional non-eating places in which you may be eating if these haven't been included.

Of course, after taking an inventory of those inappropriate non-eating places that you are eating in, you should also give yourself credit by acknowledging the ways in which you are also eating correctly by opting for the kitchen or dining room table, and other appropriate places. Using the form on page 59 as a guide, make a list below of the proper eating settings that you are utilizing on a regular basis.

Places to Eat Inventory

	Yes	No
Home		
In front of TV (couch or other seating)	_____	_____
Bedroom (bed or other)	_____	_____
Bathtub (or bathroom)	_____	_____
Garage	_____	_____
Home office (at desk or other seating)	_____	_____
Car	_____	_____
_____	_____	_____
_____	_____	_____
_____	_____	_____
At Work or School		
At your desk	_____	_____
Grabbing food at someone else's desk	_____	_____
Snacking between classes	_____	_____
_____	_____	_____
_____	_____	_____
_____	_____	_____
Other		
While working in the garden	_____	_____
While walking the dog	_____	_____
While waiting in any line	_____	_____
_____	_____	_____
_____	_____	_____
_____	_____	_____

You might have noticed that on the List of Correct Places to Eat, the word "table" is used for nearly every item (with nook or bar used in its absence). What the word "table" implies for most people is that eating is taking place while sitting down. Yes, this means eating while seated and not while standing. Eating while standing is another nonoptimal eating situation that can contribute to your eating in a manner that tends to be correlated with overeating more so than with eating in moderation. Why is that so? Well, if you think about it, typically when people are seated, particularly over a meal, they are much more relaxed and at ease, and more likely to take their time with whatever they are doing, such as consuming a meal or snack, conversing with others, or reading the paper. On the other hand, while standing, most people are more likely to feel less relaxed, in a hurry, as if they are rushing out any moment or "on the run." This can equate to a style of eating that is neither calm nor relaxed but, rather, harried, as in swallowing large gulps of not well-chewed food that is neither really tasted nor enjoyed in full. Far different from the image of someone sitting at a well-set table, complete with place mat, linen napkins, candles, and flowers (as one extreme example), is the image of someone grabbing and gulping whatever is available in the fridge. Since it is known that satiety or "fullness" tends to happen usually about 20 minutes after one has started eating, the slower and more relaxed the pace, the more inclined a person is to reach the state of fullness before it is too late, before too many calories have been ingested and undermined the weight loss effort, at least for that day.

Of course any type of weight loss surgery will facilitate a more rapid experience of satiety once eating begins, partly because the side effects of eating too much too quickly can be both extremely uncomfortable and in some cases dangerous, leading to vomiting or "dumping syndrome". But at the same time, given that weight gain post–weight loss surgery can happen in certain cases, it is still essential to learn, practice, and master all of the techniques that are typically associated with weight loss and weight loss maintenance by modifying your behavior. And on this list of techniques are both of the issues discussed above: choosing the appropriate settings and sitting down while also slowing down. In addition, because you will also be training yourself to consume very small quantities of food, it can be extremely helpful to purchase small-size plates and cups that make the food look more substantial on the plate, rather than feeling as if the meal is drowning in the plate. Part of the behavioral regimen required after surgery will also be that of allowing yourself adequate time for your meals and

List of Correct Places to Eat

	Yes	No
Kitchen table		
Breakfast nook or breakfast bar		
Dining room table		
Picnic table		
Patio table		
School dining room table		

snacks (30 minutes or more) and also planning your meals and snacks in advance, in a much more diligent way than before, to ensure adequate nutrition and such. What might be helpful for you to do, to keep track of your progress in working through these issues, is to use the checklists now to improve the behaviors that need some fine-tuning and then complete the checklists again in about six months, to see how you're doing.

Social Influences: Eating With the Right People in the Right Places

Handling certain types of challenging eating situations, such as eating at someone's home, with a group at a restaurant, at a party or celebration, at a work function, or at an event that you are hosting, can be difficult when following any type of stringent diet and perhaps even more difficult as you prepare for the type of eating you will have to do after weight loss surgery. It can even be a challenge in some instances to maintain an ongoing "eating relationship" with your family members and significant others when radical changes to your eating behaviors have taken place.

Some of the challenge depends on the specifics of the situation you are in; for instance, handling a buffet meal comes with certain advantages (you can choose your own foods) and disadvantages (the potential to eat much more than you need) as compared to a set, sit-down meal. Similarly, having an intimate meal with a small group of friends at a friend's home presents different obstacles than going to a restaurant with the same group of friends. Traveling to a foreign country will present yet another set of challenges. No matter what the circumstance, there will be times when you will have to confront eating situations that push the envelope for you—in the sense that you will be forced to be both focused on your eating plan and dietary needs, and given the options, flexible in your choices. This balance between maintaining your focus and staying flexible will ultimately prove invaluable in your long-term weight loss and weight loss maintenance efforts. To that end, it can be helpful whenever you are anticipating a challenging eating situation to do some problem solving in the session with your therapist and also in written form, to address such situations. The form on page 61 can serve as a guide.

For Teenagers

Eating at school can be challenging for teens. Usually you don't have as much time at lunch to eat, the choices available are not usually the best, and you often have to put up with a fair amount of immature, loud, and otherwise distracting behavior. Thus the school setting is conducive to quickly eating unhealthy food, in an atmosphere that is not relaxing. However, as it is generally unavoidable, it is worth the effort to try to improve the situation as much as possible. Ways to improve this include taking your lunch with the food you want and need, arranging to meet a friend or two for lunch, and finding as quiet a corner as possible to eat in.

In addition to the challenges to eating that come with the territory that you are in, the people you are with—the "cast of characters" around you during a given eating situation—can either help or hurt you when it comes to sticking with your program. As you read above in the section on social influences, there can be people in your life who are more like "coaches" and also those who are more like "saboteurs," and obviously you will want your team line-up to include more coaches than saboteurs. No matter what, it can often be helpful to have a number of catchy and clever explanations and responses at your fingertips, should the curiosity of your dining companions result in their asking a lot of questions about you, your weight loss, your food choices, and the like.

Problem-Solving Strategies for Handling Challenging Eating Situations

Challenging eating situations: _____

_____

_____

_____

Goal(s) or desired outcome: _____

_____

_____

_____

Thoughts that will help me achieve my goal: _____

_____

_____

_____

Behaviors that will help me achieve my goal: _____

_____

_____

_____

And after the fact:

Did I achieve my goal? _____ Yes _____ No

If so, why _____

_____

_____

If not, why not _____

_____

_____

Whether or not your friends and significant others know what type of diet you are on as you prepare for your surgery, they will likely begin to notice your weight loss after a given point in time. Questions will automatically follow, such as, "How did you lose so much weight?"; "Did you have the _____ surgery?" (fill in the blank with either "stomach stapling," "gastric bypass," "weight loss," or other words to describe your surgery); "Why are you eating so slowly?"; "Can you have that?"; "Should you be eating that?"; or "Don't you think you've lost enough weight?" Also there might be observations about why you are seemingly avoiding certain foods such as carbonated beverages or sweets, or comments based on a thorough or simplistic understanding of the media depiction of weight loss surgery and the behavior changes that accompany it. You will talk about your reactions to all of these questions and comments with your therapist.

In addition to these types of questions and comments, you will likely be on the receiving end of statements that are mostly complimentary in tone but that at the same time may feel intrusive, depending on the exact content and the time at which they are made relative to your beginning the process of weight loss. And of course the way any of these comments sound will depend on the source, or *who* it is that is making the comment, giving the compliment, or registering the criticism, and what your relationship with that person entails. (See earlier chapter on recording your weight, which includes a table for keeping track of weight-related compliments). For example, it would likely feel much different if a very close loved one expressed concerns about how much weight you've taken off or the rapidity of your weight loss, compared to the same sentiments when expressed by a mere acquaintance who you know very superficially.

No matter what, it is important to think about how any of these comments or questions affects you and, if necessary, to chart out the comments along with the specific thoughts, feelings, and behaviors that come up for you in reacting to what was said, similar to what was recommended in the section on compliments. The purpose of this exercise is to help you identify those external inputs that lead to unhelpful thoughts, feelings, and behaviors so that you can then challenge them using the tools previously described and other tools that you will discuss with your therapist and will read about in a later section. The form opposite can help you get started on doing that.

Comments and Reactions Log

What was said, by whom, and when:

Date	Comment(s)	Source	Reactions

As you diet to lose weight before your weight loss surgery (and eventually learn a regimen for healthy eating after), you may notice that there are certain foods that are more tempting than others and even some that are still likely to trigger urges to overeat, by a lot or a little. You may have discussed your relationship to some of these foods with your therapist, particularly if you are a binge eater who has had a problem in the past losing control over particular foods or food groups. For example, many people describe at times having cravings for salty snack foods or alternatively for sweets or chocolate. Sometimes these cravings may occur in relation to physical hunger; at other times emotions may play a larger role. Occasionally, the mere fact that the food in question is stocked at home or otherwise available might be enough to create the problem cravings. Many of the foods that you now struggle to control at times might actually invoke the feelings of a "love-hate" relationship for you based on a combination of strong cravings, a strong desire to avoid, and a not infrequent tendency to give in to the urge to lose control and overeat or binge on these foods, typically followed again by a vow to restrict their intake.

No matter what, it is important to learn both flexibility and mastery over these types of foods. For example, it might be that you are stuck at a celebration or party where only cake and ice cream—two of your most common binge foods—are being served. Whereas in the past you might either have lapsed into a bad bout of binge eating given the presence of these foods, or during a dieting episode eaten nothing at all at the party, only to binge eat on other foods later, ideally you would learn to have some of these foods in moderation, without duress. Alternatively, another solution in this type of situation would have been that of planning in advance and bringing your own healthy food to the event, if you were concerned that nothing appropriate for you would be served. That solution would be particularly important when you want to uphold the option of learning to avoid some of your challenging foods altogether, or as much as that is possible, when this may be the most reasonable strategy to follow (for example, when these foods are really threatening to your health, such as sweets if you are diabetic or specific other foods once you've had your surgery).

For some of you, depending on your own psychological and emotional issues, it might be that avoidance altogether of these certain triggering foods sets up feelings of deprivation and specific hungers or cravings that ultimately increase your likelihood for losing control when eating those foods. For example, if you are someone who has tended to overeat chocolate in the past but knows at the same time that you "can't live without it," it might be necessary to incorporate "just a little bit" at times when you are not vulnerable to overeating or losing control, to ensure that you can maintain a sense of mastery, flexibility, and control in your relationship to chocolate.

Once you have had your surgery, there will likely be certain clear-cut recommendations about foods to stay away from altogether, due to either difficulties with digestion/absorption or the ease with which these foods put weight back on you. For example, some surgery centers, or the surgeons performing certain techniques, might recommend against the intake of sweets for a year or longer (or forever) after weight loss surgery. In those instances, it may be that these foods really are "off-limits" for you and that you should learn to start living without them as soon as you can. In other instances, there may be foods that are not optimal but are acceptable as indulgences on a once-in-awhile basis. In any case, you will need to respect any of the recommendations that your surgeon has made, consistent with the general suggestions about exercising good self-care.

Incorporating Feared Foods Exercise

As you begin to think about the list of foods that you love/hate/overeat/avoid, what might work best, in addition to talking about them with your therapist, is for you to actually go to a grocery store and create a list of all of these types of "challenging foods" so that none are omitted. Once you do that, the next step is to categorize them into four different groups ranging from how easy or difficult it would be for you to experiment with eating a small or moderate portion of the food in question, that is, not fully avoiding and not overeating based on your current needs and limitations (however you define those).

This exercise should train you well, also, for the way you will have to occasionally combat your overeating habits or desires to overeat even after surgery, despite the physical limitations that the surgery imposes. You will talk more with your therapist about the "non-foolproof" aspects of weight loss surgery. For example, while any of the weight loss surgery procedures will make it much more difficult for you to overeat, and much less likely for you to *want* to overeat, the potential is still there, in particular the potential to want "just a little bit more" and to have "just that little bit"—to the point that you feel overly full or stuffed, bad about yourself, and vulnerable to overeating again in the future due in part to these bad feelings. In any case, experimenting with your intake of "feared" or challenging foods will be an exercise in mastery and flexibility over food that will generalize quite well after your surgical procedure.

Once you have created your list, use the Challenging Foods List form opposite to organize the items. You can begin to set weekly goals of eating a small amount of one or more of these foods (beginning with the least challenging and slowly working up to the more difficult foods) in settings in which you feel safe (e.g., not vulnerable to overeating because you are not "feeling fat," "out of control," or emotionally aroused or distraught in any way and because you are not in a situation in which you are likely to have access to large quantities—whatever that means to you—of the problem food). Once you have set up your eating "experiments," that is, set a goal of trying a certain food in a planned situation, try to make a commitment to follow through (except in the event of the presence of any of the vulnerability factors or danger signs for losing control noted above) and document your efforts (with a * or some other designation) in your food journal. Ideally, you will be doing such eating experiments up to a couple of times a week and in so doing will feel a great sense of liberation over any prior "extremes" in your relationship with particular foods.

For Teenagers

It is often helpful to ask parents to help you out with addressing feared foods. You can work with your therapist and parents to establish a list of foods and the situations you want to experiment with. You might decide to start off by having your parents buy and prepare the food and be with you when you try it but work up gradually to more independent experiments. In any case, you should try to use the resource your parents can be when taking this on as they can support you and be a resource to you if things don't go well.

Challenging Foods List

Group 1 (Easiest)	Group 2	Group 3	Group 4 (Most Difficult)

Homework

✎ Read the sections of this chapter on where eating happens and complete checklist.

✎ Take inventory of "people influences" on your eating and note effects of these.

✎ Work with your therapist on developing your problem-solving strategies for various eating situations.

✎ Create your feared foods list and begin to incorporate some feared foods into your meal plan.

✎ If you're a teenager, talk to your parents about feared foods and how your parents can help.

Chapter 7

Problem Solving and Cognitive Restructuring

Goals

- To help you learn methods for identifying and working through challenging problems

- To help you learn methods for identifying and working through problem thoughts

- To help you learn methods that combine problem solving and working through your thoughts so that you better handle situations that in the past might have led you either to overeating or to other nonoptimal behaviors

When faced with a dilemma of any type in which eating or overeating might have emerged as the solution in the past, in addition to the tools presented earlier (e.g., pleasurable alternative activities), you might also consider the option of engaging in formal problem solving. Problem solving is something that many people are able to do naturally and automatically, without giving it much, if any, thought at all. It might be something that you are also able to do quite easily in many, if not most, situations in which you are not stressed or overtaxed in any sense. For example, if you wake up on a given morning and it is cold and rainy as opposed to warm and sunny, you are probably able to think through your options about what to wear and to easily come up with the solution to wear warmer clothing and a raincoat, and to take an umbrella too.

If your problem-solving skills are basically good, then it is probably only in very stressful or complicated situations that you end up getting "rattled" and for that reason become confused about what you want or how to go about getting what you want. It might be that many of those stressful or confusing situations ultimately involve food in one way or another, either as the only solution that looks like it will be helpful or as a procrastination, delay, or distraction tool when a solid solution appears to be too difficult or complicated to enact straightforwardly and easily. When eating and food is used in this sense, it also serves the purpose of regulating your mood, in that it modulates any stress you might feel about the problem situation you are facing, as well as the challenge of implementing any of the complex solutions that might be warranted.

Therefore, deliberate training in and practice and rehearsal of formal problem solving is necessary to help you internalize and make as automatic as possible the process of working through even very complex and stressful problems and solutions. What formal problem solving means is engaging in a well-organized process of defining the exact problem you are facing in simple terms, brainstorming (without screening) about the possible solutions, evaluating the practicality and probable effectiveness of each solution, choosing one or a combination of these, and following through on your selected solution or combination of solutions.

The following exercise using the Problem-Solving form on page 71 can be used to help you learn the process. You should make an effort to practice this method at least a couple of times a week on various problems that you might face.

Modifying Problem Thoughts

In addition to solving certain problems or dilemmas that you might face, there are also exercises that can help you to keep your thoughts on the right track when you notice yourself slipping into problematic ways of thinking that might either lead to eating problems or other types of distress, such as emotional distress that might lead to overeating or poor self-care in general. For example, a technique called "cognitive restructuring" can be very helpful at times when you are troubled by problem thoughts. An example of this would entail a situation in which you start to feel self-conscious at a family get-together when you perceive people are watching you to see how much food you are eating because of their concern about your weight. You start to worry so much about their perceptions of you that inadvertently you find yourself overeating—simply because of the thought that keeps running through your mind: "Everyone is watching me because they think that I weigh too much to be eating so much at this meal." You realize later that although there was no actual data to objectively support your perception of your family members' views of you, you made such a strong, internal conclusion about this that you could not shake the thought from your mind and it led to a host of problem behaviors on your part (namely,

Problem-Solving

Step 1. Define the problem in simple terms: _____

_____

_____

_____

Step 2. Brainstorm about solutions (without screening): _____

_____

_____

_____

Step 3. Evaluate the practicality and effectiveness of each solution (with either "+" or "−"): _____

_____

_____

_____

_____

Step 4. Choose one or a combination of solutions: _____

_____

_____

_____

_____

Step 4. Commit to following through with your behavior: _____

_____

_____

_____

Step 5. Evaluate the entire problem-solving method: _____

_____

_____

_____

_____

negative feelings toward yourself and others and overeating) that could have been avoided if only your thought process had been a different one.

The Cognitive-Restructuring Exercise is really quite simple. All it involves is writing down the core problem thought that you have been struggling with on the top of a page and then creating two competing columns of evidence, one called "objective evidence to support the thought" and one other called "objective evidence to argue against the thought." Once you gather up all of your evidence on both sides, you should be able to come to some sort of "conclusion" that helps you modify the initial problem thought and regain your sense of clarity and calmness regarding the issue that was troubling you.

After you practice these straightforward problem-solving and problem thoughts exercises a few times, you might then try one additional spin on problem solving that combines both approaches. This technique is called the "situational analysis method" and can be used either as you anticipate a certain problem situation or after you have emerged from one, either successfully or unsuccessfully. This method involves the following: describe a problem situation that you are facing (or faced), the desired outcome that you want (or wanted), what thoughts and behaviors you should have (or should have had) onboard in order to achieve the desired outcome, and whether you achieved the outcome that you wanted. The Situational Analysis Method form (page 74) will guide you through the process. If you did achieve the outcome you wanted, describe which thoughts and behaviors were most helpful, and if not, describe how the situation actually turned out (the actual outcome) and which thoughts and behaviors were most problematic, in that they got in the way of you achieving the outcome that you wanted.

For Teenagers

Many adolescents (like some adults) are not able to use formal cognitive-restructuring techniques without a lot of therapist assistance. This is the case because cognitive restructuring requires perspective taking, generation of a range of alternatives, and the use of judgment about each option's viability and value. If you are an adolescent, you can expect that your therapist will help you to use perspective, develop alternatives, and assess alternatives, as this responsibility automatically falls to the therapist. Therapists experienced with adolescents recognize that they will need to do the groundwork on such efforts, especially at first. Therapists need to avoid "taking over" from you but will be very active in these processes with you at the start.

Cognitive-Restructuring Exercise

1. Write out the "core" problem thought in simple terms.

2. Gather up and list objective evidence to support the problem thought.

3. Do the same for objective evidence that argues against the problem thought.

4. Come up with a "reasoned conclusion" based on the evidence that will guide you to appropriate and healthy behavior

Problem Thought:

_____

_____

_____

Supportive Evidence:

_____

_____

_____

_____

Disconfirming Evidence:

_____

_____

_____

_____

Reasoned, Evidence-Based Conclusion (that will lead to positive behavior):

_____

_____

_____

_____

_____

Situational Analysis Method

Step 1. Describe the problem situation:

_____

_____

_____

Step 2. Identify the desired outcome:

_____

_____

_____

Step 3. Thoughts that will help me achieve my desired outcome:

_____

_____

_____

Step 4. Behaviors that will help me achieve my desired outcome:

_____

_____

_____

Step 5. Assess my outcome.

Did I achieve my desired outcome? If so, which thoughts and behaviors were most helpful?

_____

_____

_____

If not, what was the actual outcome, and which thoughts and behaviors got in the way the most?

_____

_____

_____

Problem solving is commonly used with adolescents when formal cognitive-restructuring strategies are too difficult or rejected. Problem solving is more direct, appeals to the immediate needs of adolescents, requires less in the way of judgment, and is experienced as being very practical. CBT therapists working with adolescents have found that problem solving is more likely to be employed with this age group than formal cognitive restructuring.

Homework

✎ Review problem solving, discuss with your therapist, and complete a few examples during the next week.

✎ Review cognitive restructuring, discuss with your therapist, and complete a few examples during the next week.

✎ Review the situational analysis method, discuss with your therapist, and complete a few examples during the next week.

Chapter 8   *Body Image*

Goals

- Help you understand the concept of body image and encourage you to discuss some of the contributions to your body image with your therapist (repeating some of the section on the CBT model)

- Increase your awareness of the issue of "body checking" and help you learn to keep frequency counts of this behavior

- Learn links between body checking and certain thoughts, feelings, and other behaviors

- Learn to identify body parts that you appreciate and that have nothing to do with weight and shape, and learn to associate these with positive thoughts, feelings, and behaviors

- Encourage use of "body image journals," capturing both the more negative and positive experiences

You might be somewhat in the dark when it comes to body image, in the sense that you might not understand exactly what it means, or you might be so resigned to concluding that your body image is defined in full by the fact that you are overweight or obese that you haven't explored the concept further. Like with issues of weighing yourself on the scale, you might simply have put your head in the sand when it comes to even *thinking* about the notion of body image.

So, first of all, what is body image? The best place to start is with a definition: body image is your internalized version of the physical realities of your body. That means, most simply, a combination of how you think and feel about your body in a long-term sense and also at any one point in time, based on the inputs of that particular situation or that moment. For example, your body image might vary somewhat even over the course of a day: before a large, holiday meal you might have a sense of feeling somewhat slim and in control of your body, and after a large holiday meal, say Thanksgiving as one example, you might have the contradictory experience of feeling "stuffed," overly large, "fat," or "bursting at the seams," particularly if any items of your clothing started to feel a bit tight after eating. Alternatively, after a long session at the gym, you might feel differently about your body, maybe experiencing yourself as relatively strong, thinner, and on the road to fitness.

If you take a few minutes here, you might be able to jot down a few words on page 79 to characterize your body image in general, as you think about it in an abstract way (e.g., not in response to a large meal, an exercise session, or a diet). It is important to take some time to reflect on the words that you write below, as likely many of these might lead to certain emotional reactions, either bad or good, some of which might even trigger episodes of eating or overeating, as discussed in earlier sections of the manual. It is likely that many of your experiences throughout your life have contributed to the way that you feel about your body, as described in part in the section on the CBT model, and you might want to keep all of those contributions in mind as you work through this chapter.

It will be important as you become more and more aware of your thoughts and feelings about your body that you discuss these in depth with your therapist, particularly as you prepare for weight loss surgery. While radical weight loss of the magnitude usually facilitated by the surgery *might* affect positive change in your body image, there is no guarantee that weight loss will lead to improved feelings about your body. Rather, it is imperative that at the same time that you are losing weight (before your surgery, if that is recommended, and after) you continue to work on underlying issues of *self-* image, which in the end are the root source of the feelings that you have about your body, whether you are obese, skinny, or somewhere in between.

In the chapter on the importance of weighing regularly and obtaining a variety of measures of your body size, shape, and general appearance (including to some extent the comments of others), you were educated about the utility of assessment of your body, that is, keeping track of where you're at. Probably, with respect to your body weight and shape, and as related to your body image, you have been doing this for some time, although you may have been quite unaware of it. Examples of how certain individuals "keep tabs" on their body (and respond with certain types of thoughts and feelings about what is happening to their body, whether positive or negative) include very common behaviors such as looking in mirrors, windows, or any reflective surfaces often; pinching various areas of the body such as

My Body Image Perceptions

the upper arms, forearms, or thighs; trying on different items of clothing to see how they might fit; and/or sitting in various pieces of furniture to see how you fit into them. If you are actively and regularly engaging in any of these behaviors, it is quite likely that you have never before given much thought to the notion of how these behaviors affect your subsequent thoughts, feelings, and behaviors. Well, now is the time to do so! As in many cases, the results of this type of checking are only negative, in terms of the effects on perceptions of the self, mood, and action (including decisions about eating and overeating).

The first place to start is to get in touch, over the course of a week or so, with exactly what you are doing to keep track of what is happening with your body by first keeping a log of what the different types of "body checking" (if any) are. You can use the form on page 81 for this task. You will eventually add some frequency counts to this data, so that you become more aware of how often you are doing what. For example, many people have been quite surprised to realize that they are pinching their upper arm to "see how fat I am" up to 20 times a day! Clearly, their weight could not have changed dramatically, if at all, within a day's time. Yet their method for continually checking by pinching themselves provided them some illusion of "staying in control" of any changes that might be happening, even though at a distance, it is clear that pinching any part of the body and weight gain can in no way be naturally correlated. Later, after this baseline data is collected, there will be an opportunity to explore more about the thoughts, feelings, and behaviors that seem to follow from these "body assessment" experiences.

Next, after discussing the above with your therapist, you will want to start keeping "frequency counts" of how many times any of these "body checks" are happening each day. The form on page 83 can be filled in with your "body checking data" as this becomes available over the next couple of weeks or so. What you will want to do as a starting place is recreate your list from page 81 in the space on page 83, and then begin to make tally marks for each of the seven days of the upcoming week, for a grand total for the week per each behavior. Ultimately, you and your therapist will discuss the importance of decreasing all types of excessive checking behavior over time, particularly as you will likely be noting its links to problem thoughts and behaviors. Therefore, over time, you will be tracking the frequencies per week and looking to see downward trajectories for each of the behaviors. Keep in mind, however, that this doesn't contradict the earlier message about the importance of weekly weighing sessions, as well as, in moderation, other

The Ways That I Check My Body

forms of "checking in" with what's happening with your body (e.g., even trying on different pieces of clothing and such). It is just the excessive checking that becomes problematic, just as problematic as denial altogether, otherwise known as "putting your head in the sand."

Next, after you discuss your "frequency data" with your therapist, you can begin to note the thoughts and feelings that seem to come up for you when you "choose" (after all, it is a choice to pay attention to a certain part of your body that represents to you your level of overweight) to focus or dwell on this area or areas. One would surmise that many of the thoughts and feelings would be more negatively toned than positive, given that the presence of body checking often implies anxiety of at least mild or moderate intensity and that the behaviors associated with those thoughts and feelings would run the gamut from avoiding people, to avoiding other positive events or experiences, to overeating (as but one nonproductive "escape route" from the negative feelings). It might be easiest and most straightforward to do this in a journal or with the form below, so that you can write about the issues freely and then have a written document to review with your therapist in your sessions. You may photocopy the form below or download multiple copies from the Treatments *ThatWork*™ Web site at www.oup.com/us/ttw.

Just to get you started, keep in mind the following "equation":

Body Checking = thoughts, feelings, additional behaviors, and maybe more body checking

In any case, once you have written down the specific thoughts, feelings, and actions that occur in relation to certain of your body-checking behaviors, you can apply one or more of the cognitive-restructuring, problem-solving, or situational analysis type of techniques to your experience, to run interference with any negative process you get into with your body-checking behaviors so that you don't work yourself into a downward spiral. For example, if you find that when you try on too many pairs of clothing in the morning, you start a downward spiral of thoughts that goes something like "I am fat, nothing fits anymore, I am going to cancel my lunch out with friends," and so on, and then you stay home and overeat on your own, it is clear that you are creating a negative experience for yourself that could be interrupted by 1) altering your thought process; 2) focusing on the problem situation at hand and identifying a desired outcome that you work toward; or 3) engaging in some type of problem-solving exercise

My Body Checking Behaviors: How Frequent Are They?

	Su	M	T	W	Th	F	Sa

in order to identify at the outset situations in which when you are vulnerable to checking your body in a way that will make you feel bad, think bad, and act badly, too.

Another issue often overwhelming to those with obesity is the basic difficulty of validating your right to experience any other aspects of your body or appearance, *other than your weight,* as important and for that reason allowing weight to play an overly significant role in determining your sense of attractiveness as a person. Therefore, it is important to help you get in touch with all of the other parts of your body and physical appearance that you might like and value, and that might even compensate at times for the way that you feel about your weight and shape, if and when you get down on yourself for carrying more weight than you need. For example, some people are able to acknowledge that they have very nice hair, hands, eyes, even feet, or a rosy, glowing complexion. Have you ever stopped to ponder the physical attributes that you have, that make you feel good about your physical self, no matter what is happening with your weight? Whether you have done this before or not, take some time to jot down a few notes about the physical features that you might also value, as you begin to put forth considerable effort to improve upon an area, your weight, that likely has been quite predominant in determining the way that you experience your physical self. Use the form on page 86 to do this exercise.

In relation to these non-weight-related body perceptions, it is equally if not even more important that you get in touch with the thoughts, feelings, and other behaviors that result from a focus on them. For example, if focusing on a "negative" such as the flab on your upper arm reminds you that you are "fat" and sets in motion a spiral of despondence, depression, isolation, and overeating, it should stand to reason that the converse would also be true, that focusing on your shiny and bouncy hair or translucent complexion would lead to feelings of well-being, contentedness, and good self-care. In the same way that you kept track of the more negatively toned body checking–related thoughts, feelings, and behaviors in the preceding minijournal, do the same with these positive experiences in the Body Image Journal on page 87. Of course, you and your therapist will take several weeks to discuss this material and undoubtedly come back to it time and again as you progress toward your surgery. It will be important at various phases after your surgery to continue to monitor your various experiences of your body image, whether "checking" per se or other associated thoughts, feelings, or behaviors, because as your body will be changing so rapidly in

Physical Features That I Like (and that have nothing to do with my weight)

Appreciated Physical Features: Related Thoughts, Feelings, and Behaviors response to the weight loss, your perceptions of your body might also become destabilized and fluctuate, possibly more during times of stress than when all else is status quo.

For Teenagers

If you are a teenager, you might find it very useful to go over these exercises with your parents and siblings. One reason to consider this is that sometimes you may not know everything you do to check your body, and a parent or brother or sister might be able to tell you. In addition, your family members might have some things to add to your positive qualities list that you haven't considered. They may also be able to help you think through some of these issues, and certainly, in conjunction with your therapists, they can provide you with a valuable perspective on your thinking and how they see it affecting what you do and how you feel.

Homework

✎ Read and discuss the chapter with your therapist.

✎ Begin self-assessment of body-checking areas and frequency counts.

✎ List out "appreciated" physical attributes.

✎ Start to work on both body image journals, the one reflecting thoughts and feelings after body checking and the one associated with thoughts and feelings about appreciated attributes.

✎ If you are a teenager, ask your family to help with these exercises to expand your perspectives and to use them for support.

Chapter 9

Congratulations! You're on Your Way to the O.R.

Goals

- ■ To orient you to all of the issues still to be addressed before your surgery

- ■ To guide you in getting in touch with deeper thoughts and feelings about your upcoming surgery

- ■ To facilitate your use of checklists and exercises pertaining to these issues

Addressing Agenda Items

No matter how much time has passed since you first began to consider a weight loss surgery procedure, as you get closer to scheduling your surgery or moving toward your actual surgery date, you will want to maintain a written list of the number of agenda items that need to be attended to before your surgery, so that all are kept "top of your mind" and none are forgotten.

Professional Consultations

Obviously, one of the most important issues here is that of having selected a weight loss surgery program that you are comfortable with and a surgeon who has agreed to work with you and perform the particular weight loss surgery procedure that you are looking for, given the options that are available to you. As part of the process of deciding on a weight loss surgery program and professional "team," you will have obtained a referral from your primary care physician and also communicated with your insurance company to determine the extent to which the array of recommended and required medical visits and treatments associated with your surgery are covered. It is likely that you, your physicians, and members of the surgical team will have completed and submitted to your insurance company a variety of forms and other paperwork to support your need for the surgery. In working with this surgeon and center, you will have been given a list of preoperative guidelines, including the required pre-op session or sessions with a mental health professional, dietician, internist, and possibly other medical personnel. And in some instances your significant other may be asked to accompany you to a given meeting.

Follow Through With Recommendations

In the context of all of the professional consultations that you will take part in, it is likely that several recommendations have been made about what you need to do to ready yourself for surgery. These suggestions might pertain to, for example, starting on a weight loss diet and exercise program or losing a given number of pounds by a certain date, or (separate from a goal of weight loss per se) eliminating or decreasing certain foods from your diet that may be problematic after surgery, adopting a specific eating schedule that is more consistent with what you will need to do post-operatively, or improving the nutritional quality of your diet. Other suggestions made during the series of evaluations may not be specifically related to weight loss. These might include participating in a support group comprised of both pre- and post-operative weight loss surgery patients that is focused on all types of issues related to the surgery; meeting with a mental health professional one or more times (in addition to the initial consultation) to work on issues of self-care, mood regulation, emotional eating, or other concerns; starting on a medication or other treatment for a condition that has been diagnosed, for instance, using a C-PAP machine to treat sleep apnea or starting on an antidepressant or mood management medication to improve or stabilize your emotional state.

No matter what the particulars, as your surgery date (or scheduling of it) draws closer, you should be "keeping tabs" on which consultation sessions have been completed and which are pending, and what you need to do to ensure that a given meeting gets scheduled. (Programs and individual practitioners may differ in terms of the expectations regarding "who contacts whom" to set up appointments and follow-up meetings.) Keeping some type of list, diary, calendar, or journal about all aspects of your surgery preparation can be helpful. (See page 91.) You might start by recording events and "to do" items on a day-by-day basis and then at the end of the

My Pre-Surgery Planning Journal

chapter, you can use the checklist provided along with your pre-surgery planning journal as you get even closer to the date.

An Introduction to Emotional and Interpersonal Readiness

Another set of issues altogether that needs to be looked at and considered seriously before surgery is that of emotional and interpersonal readiness. What this means is that you begin to think about all that the surgery means to you, in relation to, for example, following through with something you've wanted to do for yourself for some time to improve your life, while simultaneously facing the potential for certain risks and negative consequences that are always associated with radical surgery. Many different kinds of emotions can surface as you look at this layer of your experience with the surgery; for instance, you might notice feelings of guilt that you are "allowing" yourself the surgery when you're not sure you deserve it or anger that you have unfairly had to experience a weight problem to the degree that surgery is required. Likely, both anxiety and sadness, as you face the unknown of surgery and what lies ahead for you after, will be part of the picture, as well as great enthusiasm and excitement about the outcome and your new life after radical weight loss.

All of the feelings will be linked in some way to various aspects of your changing relationship with food, your body, your sense of yourself, and your relationships with other people. As you delve into all of your emotions about the surgery, you will need to stay well aware of the "opposing currents" nature of many of these changes. For example, your relationship with food will change following surgery, for both good and bad, meaning that while you will be "forced" in a sense by the procedure to adopt a more healthy relationship with food, this changed stance will also involve loss, that is, no longer having the option of using food to excess, in an attempt to soothe and comfort yourself in response to the difficult emotions or situations that you may face.

Another example of a "mixed bag" of feelings might be the bodily changes that you anticipate. While, obviously, weight loss and all that comes with it, such as improved health, mobility, and appearance, is your goal in following through with weight loss surgery, you won't be able to predict in advance what the new and thinner you will look like or how your body will "hold up" in response to the massive weight loss. Yes, your clothing sizes will eventually decrease and radically so. But certain other issues might arise in the process of losing your weight, for example, an accumulation of excess skin that doesn't shrink back after weight loss, the possibility of hernia or hair loss, and the experience of simply feeling disoriented in a physical person that you no longer recognize.

In addition to pondering all of the feelings that are likely to come up for you as you progress toward your surgery, it is also important to think about how to communicate with your loved ones about what you currently are and will be going through. You might first focus this discussion within yourself by thinking through the ways in which you can tell your loved ones and others how they can be helpful to you before, during, and after the procedure. You might also want to share with them your sense of what they could inadvertently do that might be harmful or unhelpful to you, your hopes, and your fears. And just in case the surgery does not go well—or even more remotely, in the event of death related to the surgery—you might wish to disclose thoughts and feelings you would want your loved ones to know.

The point here is not to force excessive sentimentality on you about what you will be going through but rather to have you realistically assess what is happening "inside" of you, as it relates to your upcoming surgery, and based on this what needs to be addressed "on the outside." Finding the space to do this kind of work well in advance of the surgery makes it much more likely that you can work on the issues noted previously with a clear and level head. The issues raised in the last two sections will be discussed in more detail later in the chapter.

Exercises to Access and Clarify Your Feelings About Surgery

This section will provide room for you to thoroughly examine and write about your deepest thoughts and feelings about the weight loss surgery that you are about to undergo. As you get closer to the date of surgery, you might notice that your thoughts and feelings change; thus it will be important to keep an ongoing chronicle, in journal form, of "where you are" in relation to your surgery.

Deservedness

The first exercise (opposite), entitled "Why I Am Deserving of Weight Loss Surgery and How It Will Improve My Life," provides an opportunity for you to write about why you deserve the surgery, what types of positive changes you are hoping for in undergoing the surgery, and all that you have been doing to appropriately care for yourself as you prepare for it.

Ambivalence and Concern

The second exercise might be more difficult to do. It gets back to the idea of the "opposing currents" or "mixed bag" of feelings that often come with complicated terrain like radical surgery. Specifically, it addresses the "costs" aspect of the "costs and benefits" analysis that you completed in one of the early chapters associated with undergoing the surgery. Here, it is important that you take time to think through and freely express in writing any and all of the fears, concerns, worries, or misgivings you might have about the surgery. Of course, these will differ across individuals, but the list might include attention to some of the physical risks associated with undergoing any surgery or weight loss surgery in particular, including the risk of mortality; general worries about complications, physical discomfort, or difficulties with healing; or more "trivial" worries associated with being in the hospital, finances, time away from your usual activities, and the like. By the same token, it is also essential that you get in touch with any issues of entitlement that you might have about the surgery and your recovery from it. Here, entitlement means assuming a somewhat grandiose attitude that denies any of the negative aspects potentially associated with the procedure or your recovery from it. While obviously staying positive is of the utmost importance, not blinding yourself to the potentially negative consequences of the surgery (see section immediately below) is also essential. Without keeping the door open to allow for appreciation of both the positive and the negative, you will not be appropriately prepared to take yourself and your self-care seriously at all stages of the surgical experience: preparation, initial recovery and healing, later recovery, and long-term maintenance of change. Complete Exercise 2 on page 96.

Exercise 1: Why I Am Deserving of Weight Loss Surgery and How It Will Improve My Life

Exercise 2: My Concerns About Undergoing Weight Loss Surgery

The third exercise (next page) pertains to your relationship with food and eating and how these areas of your life will be affected by the surgery. Obviously it is impossible to understand the extent to which your relationship with food will be changed by the surgery until the procedure has been done. But clearly your relationship with food and eating will be profoundly and permanently changed (with the exception of lap band surgery, which is to some extent "reversible"). While individuals become obese for different reasons—some may have a very strong familial predisposition such that, despite basically sound eating and activity patterns, obesity is a foregone conclusion, and some may have had longstanding habits of overeating or binge eating, combined with inactivity, that have caused or amplified the problem—food likely has played a significant role in their lives, if for no other reason than in response to the fact that, for good or for bad, the attention to dieting causes one to focus on eating, thereby further amplifying its importance.

Once the surgery is done, your relationship with food will have to be more "deliberate," careful and mechanical, at least at first, until the newly developed eating habits become second nature. Thus, despite the fact that the net effect of having weight loss surgery should be a decrease in appetite and a speedier route to fullness, considerable thought, at least at first, will need to be given to the experience of eating, to enable compliance with the medically necessary recommendations regarding the timing, contents, and portions of eating episodes and fluid intake. This deems one's relationship with food anything but spontaneous or "reactive" (to emotions, hunger signals, cravings, or situational factors), whereas before the surgery, many obese people would acknowledge that mostly their eating was "in response to" some type of triggering agent that often had little to do with making eating decisions that were ultimately in their best interest from a health and weight-management standpoint.

Simply stated, at least at first, food and eating will no longer have the capacity to fulfill a "recreational" purpose for you. And in this sense, there will probably be feelings of sadness, loss, frustration, or even anger, as well as a very strong need to "fill the void" left by the inability and unavailability of food to meet so many of your needs. In thinking through the earlier section on the "costs" of undergoing the surgery, it is very important to devote special attention to your altered relationship with food post-operatively and to think through how this might affect you. After this exploration, the

Exercise 3: My Relationship to Food and How It Will Change After Surgery

Exercise 4: What I Will Do to Fill the Voids Without Eating

fourth exercise (page 99) will help you focus on shifting your mind to alternative activities that don't involve food that can be at least somewhat pleasurable and gratifying (even if initially they are not as stimulating to you as food has been).

Alternative Pleasures Not Linked to Food

While it may sound superficial or simplistic to be asked the question, "what can you do instead of eat when you want to eat for reasons other than hunger," it is important to spend some time examining your response to this question. Many people who have lived for years in obese bodies have allowed issues of food and weight to predominate in their lives, such that other interests, hobbies, and relationships have literally shrunk away. Take some time to get in touch with a range of other emotionally gratifying or meaningful ways to spend your time and energy, so that you can have at your fingertips a list of reasonable alternatives to eating that make you feel interested in something, interesting, and engaged. Ideas that have worked for others include everything from taking a warm bath or shower, gardening, going for a walk, or calling a friend, to looking up information on the Internet, watching TV or a movie, and going for a short drive. In addition, specific relaxation techniques can also be helpful. Some of the standard relaxation strategies include deep breathing exercises, in which you follow a set of instructions guaranteed to help you partake in "meaningful" breathing; progressive muscle relaxation, where you tense and relax certain muscles at 30-second intervals or so, from your feet to your head; and visual imagery strategies in which you practice envisioning yourself in a restful scene, being mindful of all of the details and facets of your image that are relaxing. Instructions for breathing, progressive muscle relaxation and visual imagery can be found below.

Table 9.1 Deep Breathing Instructions

1. Sit in a relaxed position.
2. Place your hands on your lower belly.
3. Breathe in deeply so that your belly expands with each breath.
4. Imagine that you are breathing in clean, pure, beautiful air.
5. When you breathe out, feel your belly contract and picture yourself letting go of any stress or tension that you feel.

Table 9.2 Progressive Muscle Relaxation

1. Concentrate on the muscle tension you feel throughout your body.
2. Start with your lower legs. Tense your feet for 5 seconds while breathing in, and then relax as you breathe out.
3. Move up to your calves, then your quadriceps, and then your thighs, and do the same, tensing, and then relaxing each muscle group separately, coordinating your breathing as described.
4. Now focus on your lower back, stomach, and pelvis and do the same.
5. Move up to your upper back, chest, and shoulders, again tensing each group for 5 seconds and then relaxing.
6. Do the same for your hands, and then your face.
7. Finally, breathe in and tense your entire body and then relax, letting go of your breath as well as all of your tension and stress.

Handling "Coaches and Saboteurs": Yours and Others'

You have probably discovered that your relationships with the people that you are closest to in your life have already begun to change since you have made the decision to undergo weight loss surgery. Similar to others' responses to any self-care decision that you might make in your life—perhaps when you began a diet, embarked on an exciting vacation, started a new educational program, job, or relationship, or moved—their responses to your decision to undergo the surgery are likely to be, because of their own issues, biases, and agendas, quite mixed. It is important that in advance you get in touch with the stance that you want to adopt regarding your decision about and commitment to the surgery and that you also think through

Table 9.3 Visualization Exercise

1. Imagine a scene in which you feel entirely relaxed (examples that work for some people include beach scenes, taking a walk outdoors, visiting a place that has special meaning, etc).
2. Think through all of the details of your scene that enhance your feeling of relaxation such as, in the case of the beach scene, the temperature, the feeling of the sun on your skin, the smells and sounds associated with the ocean or other body of water, possibly birds flying overhead, the color of the sky and the sun.
3. Revel in each of these details as they inspire you.
4. Make sure and insert yourself into the scene, and as you enjoy the calm associated with your image, observe that you are totally relaxed, safe, and at peace.

who among your support team is likely to be more on the "coach" side and who is likely to be more on the "saboteur" side.

In considering the issues of "coach" and "saboteur," it is also important that you sort out in advance how you are likely to respond to yourself as you observe yourself going through the process of preparing for and undergoing surgery. This gets back to the issues of deservingness and also hits upon reactions of anxiety, guilt, self-sabotage, and acting out. Specifically here, you should spend time creating a mental image of yourself progressing through all of the stages associated with your surgery, from pre-op to post, keeping in mind the possibility that while all can go exceptionally well and you can emerge from surgery without complications or setbacks of any kind, it is also possible that one or more problems can occur. In the instance of an initial or later outcome that is not 100% perfect, it is important that you hold onto your commitment to feeling deserving and self-caring in all respects regarding your decision to undergo the surgery, no matter what might happen in terms of unexpected and untoward complexities that arise. This work will require that you get in touch with your deepest thoughts, feelings, and problem-solving strategies as they relate to your goals for surgery. (See Exercise 5.)

When Surgery Goes Badly: Preparing for Unlikely Complications

Finally, as you have become more and more aware of the potential benefits of the surgery, as well as the costs, the issue of mortality (death) from surgery has to be on your mind on some level. While the goal here is not to encourage you to dwell on worries about dying as the result of surgery, it is important that you come to terms with the possibility of this, no matter how remote it is, and "make peace" with yourself regarding your decision about the surgery and other aspects of your life, as well as with the significant others who are affected by all that happens in your life, including the possibility of losing you as a result of the surgery. The way that you handle getting in touch with this material by definition will be quite personal; there is no one way to approach preparing yourself and others for the remote possibility that you could die as the result of what is in most cases an elective surgical procedure. Nevertheless, the recommendation is to take some time to really think through these issues. For example, you might consider writing a letter to your significant others incorporating all that

Exercise 5: Handling Internal and External Coaches and Saboteurs

you would want to say to them, if this were your final opportunity to do so. In addition, you might want to incorporate some of the preceding material regarding your decision to have the surgery, so that they fully understand the entirety of your experience.

Also, given the likelihood that all will go well with your surgery, it is of the utmost importance to plan and prepare others to support you in the most helpful ways possible. For example, you might request certain family members or friends to provide transportation to the hospital, to stay while you are undergoing the procedure, and to be present once you wake up afterward, and so on. From others, you might request assistance in stocking your kitchen with all of the necessary foods and beverages that you will need during the first few post-op weeks. Still others might be called upon to visit you while you're at home, to provide transportation to follow-up visits and other appointments or activities, or to provide emotional assistance in the form of "a shoulder to cry on" should you need that during periods of anxiety or worry before or after the procedure. In lining up supports of this nature, essential is your ability to communicate to your significant others about your emotional state and your needs. They can't know that in addition to feeling very excited about your upcoming surgery, you are also highly anxious, worried, or struggling with guilt about "whether or not you deserve it." If you don't let people know what you are experiencing and what you need, they can't possibly respond.

For Teenagers

Obviously, if you are a teenager, your parents will be highly involved in all aspects of the pre-surgical and surgical processes. You will not be on your own. You will want to make sure that they understand the work you have done pre-surgically with your therapists and with yourself to make you (and them) confident that you can succeed. Parents always worry about their children, and yours will be concerned about protecting you as much as possible from pain and harm. However, when they have gone through the same processes you have in preparing for the surgery, they will be a great resource for you. You should try to identify how your parents can be specifically helpful to you—who will be with you when you go to the O.R., what you want waiting in the room, and how much and when you want others (friends and relatives) to know about the surgery and how you're doing afterward. Your parents will also likely be in charge of making sure all the immediate discharge medications are on the ready when you go home.

My Weight Loss Surgery Support, Supplies, and Tasks List in chapter 10 of your workbook pertains to this issue of your relationship with the important people around you.

Chapter 10

What Happens After Surgery?

Goals

◾ To help you think through the challenges you will face after surgery

◾ To facilitate your taking charge of as many of these issues as possible in advance

◾ To introduce you to CBT strategies that you can use should you experience any problems following your surgery

This chapter discusses what to expect immediately after your surgery and in the first few days and weeks that follow, and it will remind you of the importance of being fully compliant with the initial recommendations regarding your dietary intake, the amount of rest and physical activity that are optimal, and the necessity of being patient, utilizing various supports, normalizing frustrations, and so on, in the short term. In this chapter, you will be encouraged to work on various written plans of action for situations you might face after surgery. Completing these exercises, or at least thinking them through, now will enable you to be more thoughtful than you might be otherwise when facing the immediate stress of surgery or the rigors of recovery immediately after.

Once you have undergone your surgery, you deserve to give yourself a big pat on the back. You have followed through on an extensive undertaking with many mental, physical, financial, social, and logistical challenges. If you are reading this section in advance of your surgery, this section will prime you to think about the way you need to be treating yourself and the conclusion of your surgery. If you have already had your surgery, you deserve big congratulations for accomplishing your goal!

Hopefully, all will go well, or has gone well, with your procedure. At this point you are either still anticipating your surgery, or you have already undergone the procedure and are reviewing this material while recovering.

Before undergoing your surgery, it is helpful to identify those who will be able to care for you at various stages pre- and post-operatively. For example, you should have a very detailed and well-developed list of individuals who will be available for you and the specific tasks that you would like to assign to them (of course, with their permission). You will want to know well in advance who will transport you to the surgery, who will stay in the hospital while the procedure is completed, who will be there to visit you in the initial hours and up to a few days (assuming there are no complications) after, and what you would like various individuals to bring with them should you have needs of one type or another that could not be predicted in advance.

In preparing for what happens after you are discharged from the hospital, you will also want to know exactly who will "be there" for you in the hours, days, and weeks after you are at home following your surgery. For example, who will be there to keep you company, prepare any of the simple "meals" that you need, and bring those meals and fluid requirements to you? Prior to your surgery, you will want to make a detailed list of all of the food and supplies you will need. Either you or one of the members of your support team can purchase the items that will have to be on hand in the initial post-op period. Also, there may be special first aid supplies that you should have available to address any issues associated with taking care of your healing incisions. You might be prescribed certain vitamins or other medications that need to be picked up and prepared a certain way (possibly crushed, halved, or softened in some cases). Also, it is extremely important that you restart medications that you were using before surgery. Particularly important is restarting any medication related to your mood. Keeping track of all of these potential necessities, in advance of your surgery, is essential so that no detail comes as a complete surprise either for you or for those who are helping you out.

Finally, you will be having a number of required post-operative follow-up visits that are scheduled at various points after your surgery. Since it will be a matter of weeks (depending on the exact nature of the surgery) before you can drive, it is also imperative that you line up members of your support team to transport you to these visits. Obviously it goes without saying that no follow-up visit should be missed, as it is at these meetings that your surgeon and members of the team can fully assess your progress and make any suggestions, adjustments, or interventions that might be necessary.

It is at these visits that you will also be able to obtain consistent and reliable data about what is happening with your weight. While you might be one of the few who has a scale at home that has had the capacity to accurately measure your weight both before your surgery and now, usually the scales at physicians' offices are more accurate than a typical home scale, and thus you will get a spot-on reading when you see your doctor(s) at these regularly scheduled visits. The frequency and exact nature of the visits will depend on your particular surgeon and his or her program, as well as the exact nature of the surgery that you had performed. For example, open surgeries can initially require more frequent follow-up visits than laparoscopic procedures, and gastric bypass procedures more frequent visits than "lap band" procedures.

The following post-op journal and checklist (pages 110 and 111) can help you organize this information. Feel free to add as many people and tasks beyond 10 to your list as you want. You may photocopy the journal page and checklist from this book or download multiple copies at the Treatments *ThatWork*™ Web site at http://www.oup.com/us/ttw.

Assuming that the first few days out of the hospital and then at home have gone well, you might be quite relieved if not euphoric that you have made it through this very crucial initial stage of healing. Once you become aware that the first few days have passed uneventfully, it's possible that your state of mind might then shift into conjuring up the next set of worries that you might have about what you have just experienced. For example, you might become somewhat anxious about either some of your body's reactions to the surgery and/or some of the bodily changes that have already started to happen (such as continued pain in the site of the wound[s] or changes in your bathroom habits). Maybe your mind has already jumped to what the next few stages of healing, recovery, and adjustment will be like. Some people may even feel an initial, somewhat catastrophic reaction of "what have I done to myself?" that represents a type of "buyer's remorse." This type of reaction reflects anxiety about the unpredictability of what is in store and how things will progress or evolve over the next few days, weeks, and months.

While a little anxiety might be helpful to motivate someone to stay on track, too much anxiety can actually have the negative effect of shutting a person down and preventing them from caring for themselves optimally following surgery. For example, highly anxious thoughts, also known as catastrophizing, might cause a person to lose sight of the positive aspects of the decision to undergo surgery and of all of the improvements in life

My Post-Surgery Journal

My Weight Loss Surgery Support, Supplies, and Tasks List

Supplies List

1. _____
2. _____
3. _____
4. _____
5. _____
6. _____
7. _____
8. _____
9. _____
10. _____

Support Team Member	**Assignments for Him or Her**
1. _____	_____
2. _____	_____
3. _____	_____
4. _____	_____
5. _____	_____
6. _____	_____
7. _____	_____
8. _____	_____
9. _____	_____
10. _____	_____

that await the person as he or she loses weight. Instead, the person may be aware only of pain and exhaustion, stiffness and soreness, and other sensations that may accompany most radical surgeries. Or the person may choose to focus on some of the specific changes to the body caused by this surgery, for example, having a distinctly different experience of appetite that requires very extreme changes in eating habits. These physical and behavioral modifications might initially feel very scary and permanent, and thoughts like "it is always going to be like this" might occur along with worries such as "what if the surgery doesn't work and I don't lose weight"? Or "what if it wasn't worth it"?

Managing Anxious Thoughts After Surgery

It is very important that you face these anxious feelings should you experience them. It is possible to change them into thoughts that are much less worrisome and much more constructive. You will know when healthy thoughts are onboard because these will be oriented toward keeping you in an optimistic frame of mind, on the right track with respect to tasks associated with solidly recovering and healing after surgery, and focused on your commitment to learning to relate to food and your body in a new and healthier way. There are specific interventions that can help you keep your thoughts on the right track when you notice yourself slipping. You may use the cognitive-restructuring exercise from chapter 7 when you are troubled by anxious thoughts.

In addition, at such times of anxiety, when second-guessing your decision or when actually feeling some level of "buyer's remorse" during the postoperative phase, it is very important to figure out what other options you may have to quell your anxiety. While your list of pleasurable activities that don't involve food or eating will obviously be somewhat limited in the early stages after surgery (e.g., you most likely will not be able to take a bath or even a shower, or garden, exercise, or drive anywhere, much less go horseback riding or travel to Europe) you should have a short list that includes simple, relaxing, and sedentary activities such as reading, watching TV, looking up information on the Internet, chatting with a friend, and so on. It is very important to overcome any signs of anxiety in this early post-op stage because anxiety can cause you to act out—that is, engage in a behavior that is ultimately not in your best interest given your desire to heal adequately after surgery and get on with the business of serious weight loss. You might also consider the option of engaging in formal problem solving, that is, going through the process of defining the exact problem you are facing in simple terms, brainstorming (without screening) about your options, choosing one or a combination of solutions, and of course following through on your selected solution. You may wish to revisit the problem-solving exercise from chapter 7.

After at least a few weeks of adjusting to the changes associated with your surgery, you should have a sense of "how you are coming along" in terms of following through with the dietary recommendations appropriate to your post-op stage, feeling comfortable with those changes in eating, and actually losing weight. At your regular follow-up meetings with your physician, you should be obtaining feedback about how you are progressing (including documentation of your continuing weight loss) and receiving many forms of encouragement to stay on the right track; these messages should correct any misperceptions that you may have been struggling with regarding how things "should" be going as opposed to how you are actually doing, as well as any problem behaviors that you've been exhibiting. Within the first few weeks and months after your surgery, much of your focus will be on ensuring that you are handling your food and liquid intake correctly, losing weight, healing from the wounds of surgery, and generally staying positive and optimistic about all that you've been through and all that you are hoping for.

For Teenagers

Post-surgical worries of the parents of teenagers are similar to those of most patients, while an adolescent may feel less worried than many adults. So, if you're a teenager, you might want to work through some of these exercises to help not only yourself but also your parents, so that you can work together to get on with your recovery with the minimum amount of worry.

Mind and Mood

At some point within or shortly after the first couple or few months post-op, you might be ready to shift your focus from your body and all of the changes that you are going through physically to your mind and your mood.

You might even deliberately begin a process of querying yourself as to how you are really *feeling*—in an emotional sense—to get in touch with this deeper level or more subtle layer of perception (relative to body) that you might have overlooked in the flurry of activity oriented at keeping your body "on track" and healthy after surgery. While there are no established research statistics to date specifying the exact percentage of people who might develop significant, as opposed to mild, mood problems (such as depression or anxiety) at some point after weight loss surgery, there is always the possibility that a mood issue will develop. It makes sense intuitively that this may be particularly true for those individuals for whom mood issues have been present to a moderate to serious level at some point in the past, before they underwent the surgery. On the other hand, those individuals for whom mood issues were not problematic before surgery might also be affected, and again without actual data to support it, this vulnerability might be more pronounced in those who relied on food to a great degree, in the form of binge eating episodes or other compulsive eating behaviors, to regulate their mood or relied on substances or alcohol for the same effect. In any case, given the very dramatic changes to the body that happen on multiple levels following weight loss surgery, even previously nondepressed or distressed individuals might begin to feel some mood changes that are uncomfortable, and for that reason, you should be prepared to consider the possibility that this could happen to you.

Depression

In terms of "sizing up" a depressed mood, most likely what you would experience if you were falling into a depression would be at least some of the following symptoms that depressed individuals often report. These include a feeling of sadness, a sense of pessimism that is inconsistent with the positive decisions and changes you have made for yourself surrounding the surgery, tearfulness, distractibility, difficulty getting up to greet the day, difficulty performing your usual activities (any that are appropriate for your post-op stage), and in the worst cases, thoughts or plans pertaining to suicide. Clearly, if such extreme signs of depression—involving thoughts of ending your life—were present, you would likely be painfully aware of your depressed mood already, without having to do any structured form of "querying" yourself about your mood state. Rather, the depression would be "announcing itself" to you. The next steps you would take in trying to understand your mood difficulties then would involve the question of what to do to work through these problems with your mood. Mostly, it would be important to talk first to your team of professionals, including your surgeon and primary care physician; also important would be disclosing your difficulties to your trusted significant others, so that they would also know what is happening with you.

Once you let at least one, but hopefully a few, of the doctors you are working with in on the fact that you are struggling with your mood, you should rest assured that they will have a number of options at their fingertips for helping you out with respect to your depression. They might recommend that you start on an antidepressant medication, make a change to a different medication if you have been taking one with limited effectiveness, add more of something you have been taking, or restart a medication that you may have discontinued but had been taking with good effect before. In addition to discussing medications, or as an alternative to medication, psychotherapy or counseling might also be suggested, typically just involving you but possibly also at some point including a spouse, partner, or other family members.

Anxiety

Similar to depression, with respect to any anxiety problems you might be having, the issues would first be identified by your becoming a good self-observer and noting the presence of, for example, a number of persistent worries that you are having a hard time putting to rest (even with the recommended tools of cognitive-restructuring and relaxation activities and the like), ongoing muscle tension, or panic attacks. Just as with the occurrence of a depressed mood, the presence of moderate or serious anxiety would warrant your consulting with the members of your professional team, disclosing to significant others what you are going through, and thinking through, together with your "consultants," the potential viability of options such as medication, psychotherapy, and the like. Again, with only limited data to support this impression, it may be that the experience of serious anxiety by some individuals at some point post-operatively is more likely to occur in those with a history of anxiety in the past or a history of other difficulties in mood regulation that led to nonproductive solutions such as overeating and binge eating or substance use or abuse—tools that are no longer available following gastric bypass surgery, thereby leaving the individuals without easy means to assuage or "escape" the uncomfortable feelings.

Problem Eating

Another obvious category of potential problems after weight loss surgery involves that of eating. Ideally, after your surgery you will be "following the program" (in terms of all of the eating suggestions) in full, that is, eating all that is recommended, at the appropriate times and in the appropriate amounts, and drinking all that is required as well, no more, no less. In the optimal case, your following the program in this manner—that is, investing yourself fully in "doing the program right"—will yield a return on this investment rewarded by an absence of difficulties or problems. Unfortunately, even in instances in which you are doing your best to follow the program to the letter, you might experience an eating difficulty of one type or another, of an inadvertent or involuntary nature. For example, not terribly uncommon is a side effect of occasional bouts of vomiting or other gastric upsets in response to eating certain foods or, in rare instances, in response to eating anything at all. Although infrequent in occurrence, this type of vomiting might continue beyond a few episodes to become more problematic over time. In more severe cases, there could be a nutritional impact resulting from repeated vomiting episodes that builds up over time, either in the form of dehydration in the short term or even some level of malnutrition over the long term, due to not enough nutrients regularly being absorbed into the system.

There are also obvious and noteworthy physical consequences of repeated vomiting (or diarrhea, for that matter) including soreness or sensitivity in the gut or esophagus (or "lower," e.g., when going to the bathroom), as well as a psychological impact—the afflicted person might become afraid to eat due to the possibility of vomiting or experiencing "dumping syndrome" or explosive diarrhea after each and every episode of eating that is attempted. Over a period of time, this can develop into a full-blown food phobia that might look like classic anorexia nervosa to some degree, in that the affected person is likely to deny hunger or appetite, may or may not acknowledge a fear of eating, but is motivated primarily by this fear to avoid eating altogether. Clearly, if any of this seems similar to what is happening to you, it is imperative to stop the progression of this problem as early as possible by staying vigilant about your own eating patterns and habits, and feelings that may be developing in response to these. Keeping regular food records, on which you also document thoughts, feelings, situations, and the like, can be quite useful in this process of trying to understand your eating behaviors and attitudes in full. Also, taking in feedback that significant others might have for you based on their observations of your eating patterns can at times be quite helpful, even though you might initially bristle in response to what feels like judgmental control rather than helpful wisdom that can only come from outside of you. While intrusion in a situation like this is obviously not desirable, when it comes to matters like eating and mood, those around you might sometimes see more clearly what is going on for you than you are able to see yourself.

Binge Eating

A related but different problem is that of the occurrence of overeating or binge-eating episodes, obviously on a smaller scale than what would have taken place prior to the surgery. A pattern of overeating after weight loss surgery can develop slowly or insidiously over time, or might appear all of a sudden, as if out of nowhere. Again, the obvious impression one would have is that those who had problematic binge eating habits prior to surgery are more at risk for re-developing the problem after surgery (even if there was a considerable "binge free" phase before surgery was attempted) than those who never binged in the past, but so far there is no research evidence supporting this in full. In any case, a number of different types of scenarios involving overeating might develop over time in a post-op weight loss surgery patient. For example, in one individual, a craving for "just a little bit" of a certain type of food might trigger the beginning of what ultimately becomes an overeating episode, at least overeating from the standpoint of what is ideal in terms of food contents and quantities that are recommended after weight loss surgery (even if this exact eating episode would have been considered perfectly acceptable before surgery). At the point when the eating episode transitions from normal or acceptable to problematic, the person involved might also start producing a number of problematic cognitions that might make it more likely that the individual ends up eating more in response to this initial bit of overeating rather than stopping when he or she still can. This represents an example of the type of "catastrophic" thinking described earlier in this chapter. For example, entertaining a thought that goes something like, "Now I've gone and blown it! I am ruining my surgery and will never lose weight!" would obviously be more likely to perpetuate additional problematic behaviors than to curtail all of these that have just started to happen, at their earliest stages.

Cravings

Another type of overeating or binge episode that might happen "out of the blue" would involve an individual developing a strong craving for a particular food. Thinking optimistically and in the direction of good self-care that can sometimes involve "indulgence in moderation," the individual might allow him- or herself a "treat" of some type and then end up having an experience characterized as "my eyes were bigger than my stomach." What this means is that in their zeal to take in as much of the "really good indulgence food" that they want or "can" consume, a person ends up significantly overeating relative to the post–weight loss surgery recommendations. Some in this instance might go on to experience "dumping syndrome" in response, partly depending on the amounts and types of foods that were ingested, which results in stomach upset at minimum and sweating, trembling, diarrhea, and possibly vomiting as potentialities. In this instance, as much as the "dumping syndrome" proves to be a negative reinforcer for overeating, that is, maximizing the distress or negative consequence that results from overeating to the point that many would then be tempted to avoid it at all costs, some may ultimately experience the "dump" as something akin to a "purge." When it is seen this way, as a purge that eliminates food from the body, it enables the person to feel—even if illogically—that they have in essence rid themselves of the excess food and calories consumed and therefore can do it again if and when they feel like it. (This is the same logic that keeps bulimic individuals tied to their habit of binge eating and purging.)

If overeating in this fashion has been a problem for the person in the past, there may be a greater likelihood of a pattern developing yet again, particularly if there have been mood effects associated with all stages of the binge and purge cycle (for example, an initial anxiety, followed by a distracted euphoria, followed by panic, followed by discomfort, followed by calm) linked to the cycle of overeating. In all such instances of repeated bouts of problematic eating of this nature occurring over time (repeated being more than a "few" in a week or a few weeks' time), it is absolutely essential that the affected individual (that is YOU) seek professional attention as soon as possible. The starting point for this would again be consulting with your primary care physician and surgeon, so that they are apprised of the problem behavior. Their involvement is particularly important since they know what to look for in terms of any potential physical damage or side effects and know to whom to refer you for appropriate care. In the case of binge eating along the lines of what was described here, therapy with an eating disorders expert who might also recommend a consultation with an appropriate physician for some type of medication that might help to control the eating behavior and any mood contributions are likely the treatment(s) of choice, along with utilization of all of the other supports, including significant others and support group meetings.

Alcohol and Drugs

Finally, one other cluster of problematic behavior patterns that can occur after any type of stressful life experience such as that of radical surgery is abuse of alcohol or drugs. Again, those with predispositions for this type of problem, based on a family history of substance abuse or more likely their own history of any type of substance abuse occurring even years before undergoing the surgery (as stated earlier in this manual, most programs require that patients are "clean and sober" for at least 5 years before going through weight loss surgery), are probably more at risk than others who have had no experiences abusing or developing a dependency on any type of substances. However, in a manner that is similar to the development of the problematic eating behavior, these issues might develop secondary to the existence of an as yet untreated, underlying mood disorder, such as anxiety or depression. Clearly, obtaining speedy and adequate treatment for any mood regulation problems you might be having after your surgery likely decreases the probability that you will rely on these other inappropriate strategies for managing your mood, for instance, misuse of food, drugs, or alcohol. However, if you do notice any type of substance abuse problems developing or resurfacing at any point after your surgery, the same recommendations apply: you need to seek professional assistance as soon as possible. You should not, by the way, under any circumstances, concern yourself in any of these instances with problematic thoughts that pertain to feeling as if you have "let down" the members of your surgical or medical team or that you have "broken the rules" or will be "getting in trouble." The simple fact of the matter is that you are in acute need of professional assistance, and the sooner you are able to get help, the better off you will be.

Options for Seeking Help

In all of the instances noted above—involving mood, eating, and substance abuse issues—the problems were serious enough to warrant and require individual professional assistance. Keep in mind, however, that *any* type of problematic feeling or behavior, no matter how mild, deserves in and of itself some type of attention and treatment. So don't interpret the above to mean that "unless my problem is severe and includes depression, anxiety, major eating issues, or substance abuse, I should not seek help." The reality is, even if you are doing amazingly well or moderately well with the exception of a few minor problems, if you want extra help or assistance, either in the form of individual psychotherapy (that may or may not include a consultation for medications), couples counseling, or group interventions—either AA (Alcoholics Anonymous) or OA (Overeaters Anonymous), in addition to your weight loss surgery support group, or any other type of group forum—you should feel that you are healthfully entitled to seek it out. In terms of individual therapy, most important may be the "chemistry" or fit between you and the individual therapist assigned to you. By the same token, there are several different "schools" of individual therapy that you might educate yourself about, albeit somewhat superficially, just to know what the options are.

Cognitive Behavioral Therapy

Cognitive behavioral therapy (CBT) in a most basic sense would address the types of thoughts you are having and behaviors you are exhibiting relative to issues of your surgery, eating, weight, body shape, and other concerns. The sessions would likely be somewhat structured and driven by an "agenda" that is based on yours and the therapist's ideas about appropriate goals for the stage of therapy that you are in. In CBT, you are often assigned homework at each session, so that your between session time is like a laboratory in that you are encouraged to experiment on various new perspectives and behaviors you have been talking about in your sessions.

CBT Self-Help Manuals

This is a "shorthand form" of CBT therapy based on a written manual, used in conjunction with intermittent and brief (e.g., every other week, 20 minutes each) therapy sessions that are oriented toward keeping you focused on the tasks and issues presented in the book.

Interpersonal Therapy

Interpersonal therapy (IPT) is a less directive approach to treatment, although there is a clearly defined agenda that involves you talking about one or a few primary interpersonal problem areas of your life, for example, navigating a difficult transition, such as that associated with becoming thin for the first time ever (or the first time in a long while), or experiencing conflicts with other people on a very frequent basis. In the initial few sessions of IPT, you might take some time to reflect on your entire social life, the number, quality, and type of relationships you have, and have had, in an attempt to identify the core problem areas that are troubling to you. In many cases, it turns out that these same problem areas have also been instrumental to one degree or another in triggering or perpetuating aspects of your disordered eating behavior in the past, whether overeating, binge eating, or exhibiting any other form of eating problem.

Other Therapies

Many other types of therapy exist and are practiced in a form that could potentially be very helpful for someone with an eating disorder. These days, emotion regulation therapy, in which you are taught a number of different strategies and tools to embrace, validate, modify, and gently nudge toward change any excessive or nonconstructive emotional reactions you may have in a variety of different situations, has become quite popular, particularly in the treatment of all types of eating disorder issues. And there are several "nonspecific" therapies that may offer support, encouragement, feedback, reality checks, and an opportunity for accountability that can be quite helpful if delivered by the right person, to the right person, in the right circumstance. In any event, given the significance of what you have been through, in terms of following through with your surgery after a long period of preparation and anticipation, psychotherapy or counseling, just to have "someone in your court" (in the form of a psychotherapist or counselor) who is supportive, objective, there for you, and hopefully a source of wisdom and guidance, might be something for you to consider if you have any interest in it at all.

Homework

✎ Complete the exercises in this section.

✎ Take some time to relax! (Use progressive muscle relaxation, breathing exercises, items on your list of alternative activities that don't involve food, or anything else.)

References

Agras, W. S., & Apple, R. F. (1997). *Overcoming eating disorders: A cognitive-behavioral treatment for binge-eating disorder, Client Workbook.* New York: Oxford University Press.

American Medical Association. (2003). *American Medical Association roadmaps for clinical practice: Assessment and management of adult obesity, a primer for physicians.* Chicago: Author.

American Psychiatric Association. (1994). *Diagnostic and statistical manual of mental disorders* (4th ed.). Washington, DC: Author.

Arnow, B., Kenardy, J., & Agras, W. S. (1992). Binge eating among the obese: A descriptive study. *Journal of Behavioral Medicine, 15,* 155–170.

Bacon, L., Stern, J.S., Van Loan, M. D., & Kleim, N. L. (2005). Size acceptance and intuitive eating improve health for obese, female chronic dieters. *Journal of the American Dietetic Association 105*(6), 929–936.

Barlow, D. H. (2004). Psychological treatments. *American Psychologist, 59*(9), 869–878.

Bocchieri, L. E., Meana, M., & Fisher, B. L. (2002). Perceived psychosocial outcomes of gastric bypass surgery: A qualitative study. *Obesity Surgery, 12*(6), 781–788.

Bruce, B., & Agras, W. S. (1992). Binge eating in females: A population-based investigation. *International Journal of Eating Disorders, 12,* 365–373.

Buchwald, H., Avidor, Y., Braunwald, E., Jensen, M., & Pories, W. (2004). Bariatric surgery: A systematic review and meta-analysis. *Journal of the American Medical Association, 292*(14), 1724–1737.

Buddeberg-Fischer, B., Klaghofer, R., Sigrist, S., & Buddeberg, C. (2004). Impact of psychosocial stress and symptoms on indication for bariatric surgery and outcome in morbidly obese patients. *Obesity Surgery, 14*(3), 361–369.

Burns, David D. (1990). *The feeling good handbook.* New York: Plume Press.

Cash, Thomas F. (1997). *The body image workbook: An 8-step program for learning to like your looks.* Oakland, CA: New Harbinger Press.

Colquitt, J., Clegg, A., Sidhu, M., & Royal, P. (2005). Surgery for morbid obesity. *The Cochrane Library Database, No. 3,* CD003641.

Dansinger, M. L., Gleason, J. A., Griffith, J. L., Selker, H. P., & Schaefer, E. (2005). Comparison of the Atkins, Ornish, Weight Watchers, and

Zone diets for weight loss and heart disease risk reduction: A randomized trial. *Journal of the American Medical Association, 293*(1), 43–53.

Delin, C. R, Watts, J. M., & Bassett, D. L. (1995). An exploration of the outcomes of gastric bypass surgery for morbid obesity: Patient characteristics and indices of success. *Obesity Surgery, 5*(2), 159–170.

Dement, W. C., & Vaughan, C. (2000). *The promise of sleep: A pioneer in sleep medicine explores the vital connection between health, happiness, and a good night's sleep.* New York: Bantam Dell.

DiLillo, V., Siegfried, N. J., & Smith West, D. (2003). Incorporating motivational interviewing into behavioral obesity treatment. *Cognitive and Behavioral Practice, 10,* 120–130.

Fairburn, C. (1995). *Overcoming binge eating.* New York: Guilford Press.

Greenberg, I., Perna, F., Kaplan, M., & Sullivan, M. A. (2005). Behavioral and psychological factors in the assessment and treatment of obesity surgery patients. *Obesity Research, 13,* 244–249.

Grilo, C. M., Masheb, R. M., Brody, M., Burke-Martindale, C. H., & Rothschild, B. S. (2005). Binge eating and self-esteem predict body image dissatisfaction among obese men and women seeking bariatric surgery. *International Journal of Eating Disorders, 37*(4), 347–351.

Grilo, C. M., Masheb, R. M., Brody, M., Toth, C., Burke-Martindale, C. H., & Rothschild, B. S. (2005). Childhood maltreatment in extremely obese male and female bariatric surgery candidates. *Obesity Research, 13,* 123–130.

Harter, S., Bresnick, S., Bouchey, H. A., & Whitesell, N. R. (1997). The development of multiple role-related selves during adolescence. *Development and Psychopathology, 9,* 835–853.

Hay, P., & Bacaltchuk, J. (2004). Bulimia nervosa. *Clinical Evidence, 12,* 1326–1347.

Hepertz, S., Keilmann, R., Wolf, A. M., Hedebrand, J., & Senf, W. (2004). Do psychosocial variables predict weight loss or mental health after obesity surgery? A systematic review. *Obesity Research, 12,* 1554–1569.

Holzwarth, R, Huber, D., Majkrzak, A., & Tareen, B. (2002). Outcome of gastric bypass patients. *Obesity Surgery, 12*(2), 261–264.

Hsu, L. K. G., Betancourt, S., & Sullivan, S. P. (1996). Eating disturbances before and after vertical banded gastroplasty: A pilot study. *International Journal of Eating Disorders, 19*(1), 23–34.

Hsu, L. K. G., Mulliken, B., McDonagh, B., Krupa Das, S., Rand, W., & Fairburn, C. G., et al. (2002). Binge eating disorder in extreme obesity. *Journal of Obesity, 26*(10), 1398–1403.

Hsu, L. K. G., Sullivan, S. P., & Benotti, P. N. (1998). Eating disturbances and outcome of gastric bypass surgery: A pilot study. *International Journal of Eating Disorders, 21*(4), 385–390.

Huddleston, P. (1996). *Prepare for surgery, heal faster: A guide of mind-body techniques.* Cambridge, MA: Angel River Press.

Institute of Medicine (2001). Crossing the quality chasm: A new health system for the 21st century. Washington, DC: Institute of Medicine.

Livingston, E. H., Huerta, S., Arthur, D., Lee, S., De Shields, S., & Heber, D. (2002). Male gender is a predictor of morbidity and age a predictor of mortality for patients undergoing gastric bypass surgery. *Annals of Surgery, 236*(5), 576–582.

Livingston, E. H., & Ko, C. Y. (2002). Assessing the relative contribution of individual risk factors on surgical outcome for gastric bypass surgery: A baseline probability analysis. *Journal of Surgery Research, 105*(1), 48–52.

Maggard, M. A., Shugarman, L. R., Suttorp, M., Maglione, M., Sugerman, H. J., Livingston, E. H., et al. (2005). Meta-analysis: Surgical treatment of obesity. *Annals of Internal Medicine, 142,* 547–559.

McCullough, James P., Jr. (2000). *Treatment for chronic depression: Cognitive behavioral analysis system of psychotherapy* (CBASP). New York: Guilford Press.

National Institutes of Health & National Heart, Lung, and Blood Institute. (1998). *Clinical guidelines on the identification, evaluation, and treatment of overweight and obesity in adults: The evidence report.* Bethesda, MD: National Institutes of Health.

Pope, G. D., Birkmeyer, J. D., & Finlayson, S. R. (2002). National trends in utilization and in-hospital outcomes of bariatric surgery. *Journal of Gastrointestinal Surgery, 6*(6), 855–861.

Powers, P. S., Perez, A., Boyd, F., & Rosemurgy, A. (1999). Eating pathology before and after bariatric surgery: A prospective review. *International Journal of Eating Disorders, 25,* 293–300.

Sarwer, D. B., Wadden, T. A., & Fabricatore, A. N. (2005). Psychosocial and behavioral aspects of bariatric surgery. *Obesity Research, 13,* 639–648.

Shuster, M. H., & Vazquez, J. A. (2005). Nutritional concerns related to Roux-en-Y gastric bypass: What every clinician needs to know. *Critical Care Nursing Quarterly, 28*(3), 227–260; quiz 261–262.

Smith, D. E., Marcus, M. D., & Kaye, W. (1992). Cognitive-behavioral treatment of obese binge eaters. *International Journal of Eating Disorders, 12,* 257–262.

Striegel-Moore, R. H. (1993). Etiology of binge eating: A developmental perspective. In C. G. Fairburn & G. T. Wilson (Eds.), *Binge eating: Na-*

ture, assessment, and treatment (pp. 144–172). New York: Guilford Press.

Tsai, A. G., & Wadden, T. A. (2005). Systematic review: An evaluation of major commercial weight loss programs in the United States. *Annals of Internal Medicine, 142*(1), 56–66.

Wadden, T. A., Sarwer, D. B., Womble, L. G., Foster, G. D., McGuckin, B. G., & Schimmel, A. (2002). Psychosocial aspects of obesity and obesity surgery. *Surgical Clinics of North America, 81*(5), 1001–1024.

Woodward, B. G. (2001). *A complete guide to obesity surgery: Everything you need to know about weight loss surgery and how to succeed.* New Bern, NC: Trafford Publishing, 2001.

Yanovski, S. Z. (1993). Binge eating disorder: Current knowledge and future directions. *Obesity Research, 1,* 306–324.

About the Authors

Robin F. Apple received her PhD from the University of California–Los Angeles in 1991 and has published articles and chapters in the area of eating disorders. She has also cowritten a patient manual and a therapist guide that utilize cognitive-behavioral therapy (CBT) techniques for treating bulimia nervosa and binge eating disorder. In her current role as associate clinical professor, Department of Psychiatry and Behavioral Sciences, Stanford University, she has completed over 500 pre-operative evaluations of patients seeking weight loss surgery, has co-led a weight loss surgery support group, and has provided short- and long-term individual therapy for those preparing for and adjusting to their surgery. Apple maintains a varied caseload of patients with eating disorders and other issues, both at Stanford and in her private practice in Palo Alto, California. She consults on weight loss surgery–related research and forensics cases and is actively involved in Stanford's training program for postdoctoral psychology fellows and psychiatry residents.

James Lock, MD, PhD, is associate professor of child psychiatry and pediatrics in the Department of Psychiatry and Behavioral Sciences at Stanford University School of Medicine, where he has taught since 1993. He is board certified in adult, as well as child and adolescent, psychiatry. In the Division of Child Psychiatry and Child Development, he is currently director of the Eating Disorders Program that consists of both inpatient and outpatient treatment facilities. His major research and clinical interests are in psychotherapy research, especially in children and adolescents, specifically for those with eating disorders. In addition, he is interested in the psychosexual development of children and adolescents and related risks for psychopathology. Lock has published over 100 articles, abstracts, and book chapters. He is the author, along with Daniel le Grange, Stewart Agras, and Christopher Dare, of the only evidence-based treatment manual for anorexia nervosa, called *Treatment Manual for Anorexia Nervosa: A Family-Based Approach*. He has also recently published a book for parents, *Help Your Teenager Beat an Eating Disorder*. He serves on the editorial panel of many scientific journals especially focused on psychotherapy and eating disorders related to child and adolescent mental health. He has lectured widely in the United States, Europe, and Australia. Lock is the recipient of a National Institute of Mental Health (NIMH) Career Development Award and an NIMH Mid-Career Award, both focused on enhancing psychosocial treatments of eating disorders in children and adolescents. He is the principal investigator at Stanford on a National Institutes of Health–funded multisite trial comparing individual and family approaches to anorexia nervosa in adolescents.

Rebecka Peebles, MD, is an instructor in adolescent medicine at the Department of Pediatrics at Stanford University School of Medicine. She completed her training at the Cleveland Clinic Foundation and at Stanford University School of Medicine, and is board certified in pediatrics and in adolescent medicine. She is a member of the Adolescent Bariatric Surgery Board and works in the Eating Disorders Clinic and the Pediatric Weight Clinic at Lucile Packard Children's Hospital at Stanford. Her major research and clinical interests are in health outcomes of binge eating and purging behaviors, and in better understanding links between eating disorders and obesity. In addition, she has researched the impact of the Internet and pro–eating disorder Web sites on adolescent populations. She is the recipient of multiple awards for teaching and humanistic medicine. She has written on eating disorders and obesity, and frequently lectures on these topics and adolescent health in the community.